What People are Saying:

This is the story of one devoted husband's journey with his wife as his partner and ultimately her caregiver, richly informative, told with compassion and transparency as he shares his journey of denial, acceptance, loss, grief, suffering and healing. His poignant descriptions of the signposts along the way, the challenges and stress – embracing the difficult decisions regarding home care and end-of-life issues are rich with humility, compassion and love.

Catherine R. Judd Caregiver and Educator
Clinical Assistant Professor at the Southwestern School of Health Professions

Richard and Thelma's story tells what it is like to travel with someone thru the disease of Alzheimer's. Even though everyone's journey is unique, we all share similar emotions and walk thru the different stages of the disease with similar difficulties. The thought-provoking questions at the end of each chapter help the reader to relate their story to Richard and Thelma's in a personal way. Thank you to Richard for putting in writing his journey.

Marylynne Henry caregiver
Friends Place Adult Day Services, DeSoto, TX

As a music therapist, I have had many opportunities to work with memory care residents / patients. It is always rewarding to see many of them come alive when they hear music from their past. I'm
this book, from another perspe
help for many caregivers who

D1212636

deal with the unknowns of this dread disease."
Joseph Linn MA, MT-BC, Music Therapy

Richard Blake's book *Our Journey with Alzheimer's...*
is more than a touching memoir. It is an instruction
manual for those who face this dreaded disease. My
friend and fellow writer has produced a valuable and
memorable guide.
Nan Baker Author

Richard Blake writes like he lives -- with warmth,
kindness, love, and sensitivity. His commitment to walk
with care beside his wife in the Alzheimer's tunnel will
inspire and encourage other families for sure.

This is a tender, detailed memoir, destined to come
alongside many on the same journey.
Knute Larson Pastoral coach
Pastor emeritus, The Chapel, Akron

I wish your book had been available when my family
faced my father's Alzheimer's. I particularly like your
describing and organizing your experiences through the
Seven Stages categories (It makes the decline more
understandable.) and your emphasis on maintaining
caregiver health.
S.M. Kozubek Attorney

Our Journey with Alzheimer's is a must read for
everyone. Caregivers often walk this road alone, with
family and friends not understanding the emotional
roller coaster in a caregiver's day. A caregiver, along
with others, may be in denial in the early stages of
Alzheimer's. However, soon reality sets in when the
primary caregiver can no longer deny there is a lack of
capacity in his or her loved ones' actions. To other
family members and friends, this is not always evident

and denial is exhibited. Walking in someone's shoes makes a difference. This book gives light to what it is like 'walking in a caregiver's shoes.' *Our Journey with Alzheimer's* is for family, friends, church staff, work colleagues, etc. as you are taken chronologically into the home of a husband dedicated to his wife's care, while experiencing emotions he would have never thought.
Carolyn Legg MS, CSA, CMC, CDP
Caregivers Connection 4U, LLC
Geriatric Care Management 4U, LLC

I hope you savor this love story penned by my good friend, Richard Blake, including the relentless, downward spiral of his dear wife, Thelma, as she slides into the abyss of confusion and forgetfulness. You will be moved and gain numerous insights as the couple lives through each season of "Seven Stages of Alzheimer's." No easy answers, just real life frustration, fear, laughter, uncertainty, puzzlement, faith, and final celebration throughout the couple's brave encounter with the "A" word that enslaves 5+ million fellow citizens. Kudos, Dick, for candor and grace, story-telling skill, and for including us on the journey.
Pastor John Bedford

Our Journey with Alzheimer's is a great insight to the challenges and emotional stressors Caregivers face. It depicts the kind of love, commitment and friendships needed to travel this road. This read is enlightening. It will make you smile, cry and appreciate your loved ones.

Belyne Bland-Xochihua LBSW, MPH
Medical Social Worker

OUR JOURNEY WITH ALZHEIMER'S

OUR JOURNEY WITH ALZHEIMER'S

SIXTY-FIVE YEARS OF LOVE AND COMMITMENT

INSIGHTS FOR FAMILY CAREGIVERS

RICHARD R. BLAKE

ISBN 978-1-7358145-2-0

Dedication

I dedicate this our story to my wife, Thelma, my princess and the joy of my life and to our four sons, Rick, Ken, Jim and Rob, whose love, respect and encouragement has blessed us on our journey.

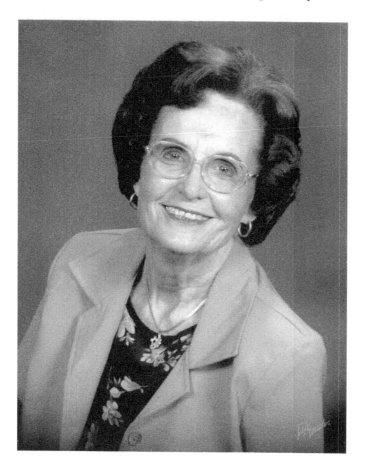

Acknowledgements

I want to acknowledge my gratitude to God who was right there with me through our journey and who continues to sustain me day by day.

I want to express my appreciation to the pastors, staff, and friends, at Redwood Chapel Community Church in Castro Valley, California and Woodland Shores Baptist Church in Bridgman, Michigan for their spiritual impact on us individually and as a family.

I want to express gratitude to family, friends and caregivers (too numerous to mention by name) who helped Thelma and I through this long journey. I never could have done it without you.

I am deeply grateful to staff at Woodland Terrace as well as the Bridgman Alzheimer's Support Group. who shared the last five years of our journey.

I also want to thank Jon Drury and the Castro Valley Writers Group as well as the Bridgman Library Writers Group for encouraging me in writing the story of our journey.

A special thanks goes to my sister, Edna Headland, who has diligently led me step by step in the editing process. We spent many hours together on ZOOM while she shared her screen piecing together my story as I gathered recorded remembrances, notes, and journals of over sixty-five years. She helped me realize my dream by gently prodding me to keep going. Her understanding of Alzheimer's Disease as a nurse and the impact on the caregiver gained through participation in Caregiver's groups made her input invaluable in formulating the *Questions for Reflection or Discussion*. She has been an inspiration to me through her example of Christian service with Wycliffe Bible Translators for nearly sixty years. I shared in the process of writing her book *His Grace is Sufficient: Bible Translation with the Tunebo of Colombia.*

Contents

Foreward

It is my honor to write a word of endorsement for "Our Journey with Alzheimer's." As a professional speaker and trainer with a background in memory care development, it is always a blessing to discover rich resources which can help others who are experiencing their own battle with this disease.

This is a well written true story, full of relatable life experiences, ultimately leading the writer and his wife to and through the long and difficult journey of Alzheimer's disease.

Their love story speaks for itself. The reader is drawn into the story of Richard and Thelma's personal and professional intersections of family life and ministry across the years.

With merely a hint to what lies ahead on their journey, the writer piques interest in the reader to imagine their own possible response to what is extremely difficult to accept, the insidious disease of Alzheimer's which is no respecter of people at any stage of life. No matter who has it or how long it takes to recognize the fullness of its impact, this disease simply doesn't stop... for anyone. The toll on families especially family caregivers is undoubtedly one of the most difficult aspects of the disease.

I found the book to be a great reference with many tips and insights needed to understand the depth of the disease. It is full of relevant examples to enhance understanding. In reading each chapter, I was moved as I was reminded that "nothing teaches like experience", a lesson none of us wants to learn in relationship to this disease.

A unique offering in this book, is a series of *Questions for Reflection or Discussion* which heighten the reader's awareness of the disease process and develop a better understanding of what can be anticipated on the path ahead. In my opinion, this portion of the book is very beneficial in gaining more clarity on many aspects of the disease, giving caregivers a guide for further discussion.

This book provides a tender look at the unique acceptance found in the writer's personal faith and intimate knowledge of the Lord's guiding hand through each stage of his wife's illness. The writing inspires the reader to evaluate their own response to trusting God in the most difficult of circumstances.

I admire the clarity with which the author shares the deep impact of Alzheimer's and the ultimate cost in which families affected must share. Richard's deep love for his wife, evidenced by his tender, compassionate and servant hearted care and his abiding trust in God's provision at every turn, bears witness to the power of love as the ultimate healer, regardless of what any disease is called.

If you or a loved one is facing Alzheimer's disease "head on," I recommend this book without reservation.

Rev. Marti Miller
ADC. CALM. CDP. CADDCT. CDCM

Introduction

As of the end of 2019 the number of Americans living with Alzheimer's is growing — and growing fast. An estimated 5.7 million Americans have Alzheimer's disease. Alzheimer's disease research estimates that every 65 seconds someone in America develops the disease.[i]

An alarming statistic not noted above is the fact that additionally thousands of those impacted by the disease will be family caregivers; children and spouses.

Our Journey with Alzheimer's includes notes from my journal, stories, our experiences, and lessons we have learned over the 24 years of our journey.

Alzheimer's support groups have been a tremendous help to me, as a caregiver. I have included *Questions for Reflection or Discussion* to help other caregivers process their experiences. They can be used either for reflection by the individual reader or for discussion in a caregiver's group.

The book is divided into three parts: Part 1 Life Before Alzheimer's, Part 2 The Seven Stages of Alzheimer's, Part 3 Afterwards.

For the Purposes of this book we have used the Seven Stages of Alzheimer's Disease, developed by Dr. Barry Reisberg of New York University.[ii]

Richard R. Blake

Part One
Life Before
Alzheimer's

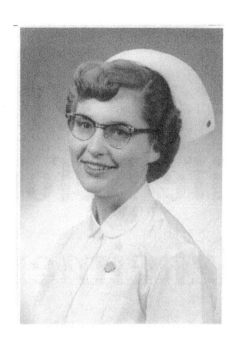

Thelma as a young nurse

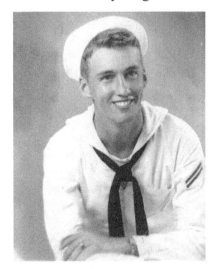

Richard in the Navy

Courtship and Marriage

Love at First Sight

I was at the piano, with more nerve than talent, I missed another note, the singing went right on, but I was distracted, I heard a buzzing of voices, quiet whispers, and the shuffling of chairs being added to make room for latecomers.

As the song ended, I turned around on the bench, our eyes met, and she smiled. I melted. Third row back, her eyes sparkled as her smile widened. I was hooked.

After another song, I left the piano bench to take a seat angled in a way that gave me a clear unobstructed, view of the student nurse with the sparkling brown eyes and the million dollar smile. Her name was Thelma Barnes, a first-year student at the Samuel Merritt School of Nursing in Oakland.

Tonight was the first in a series of training sessions for volunteer prayer room counselors. We were to be participating in the Saturday night Youth for Christ (YFC) evangelistic rallies, held in the Oakland Auditorium.

In the 1950s, Youth for Christ was nationally recognized by evangelical churches for their youth emphasis in high school clubs and weekly evangelistic rallies.

Counselors were to be ready to encourage those who responded to an invitation to follow Christ. Those who responded were escorted to a prayer room to affirm their decision. As counselors we were assigned seats at the back of the auditorium.

21

The following Saturday evening in September my eyes scanned the auditorium as I joined the crowd looking for their seats. When I found my reserved seat, imagine my surprise and delight – you guessed it – the girl named Thelma was assigned the one next to mine.

The Saturday night rallies, the social hour at the YFC Servicemen's Center after the rally, and the training session on Monday nights made it possible for Thelma and me to see each other two nights a week without really dating. By fate, divine providence, or the luck of the draw Thelma was also in the interactive group I facilitated as a part of the counselor training.

Christmas Banquet – Our First Official Date

Four months later, in December the Youth for Christ leadership arranged a Christmas banquet at the historic Claremont Hotel in Berkeley. I worked up the courage to ask Thelma to be my date for the event.

I was dressed in my freshly cleaned blue uniform and "spit-shined" shoes when I picked up Thelma at the Farley Hall dormitory. Thelma was strikingly elegant in her black taffeta dress with small pink flowers. The abundance of petticoats worn in the fifties filled out the skirt accentuating Thelma's tiny waist. I presented her with a pink carnation corsage. My chest inflated with pride as I walked her to the car. We were double dating with our friends Glenn and Beverly Morrison.

Nestled in the hills of Berkeley, overlooking the San Francisco Bay, the twenty-two acres of natural grounds gave the Claremont a timeless setting and a picturesque historic charm. As we walked through the lobby of the Claremont, I looked up at the sparkling chandeliers. They glittered like cut diamonds. I gawked upward like a farm boy at the splendor of the décor. As we walked down the deeply carpeted stately circular staircase to the dining room on the lower level, we could see the lights of San Francisco on the other side of the bay.

Thelma's eyes added sparkle to the reflection of the chandeliers, flickering candles, and crystal glasses. We were awed throughout the evening. The food, the service, and the program all contributed to making this, a never to be forgotten first, in a series of many memorable dates over the next 65 years.

Thelma never lost that sparkle, or spontaneous affection for people; always radiating love and an enthusiasm for life.

A Still Small Voice

Five months later we walked from Telegraph Avenue along 34th Street to Farley Hall, Samuel Merritt Hospital student nurse's dormitory. As Thelma and I walked, my hand found Thelma's, she smiled. I thought we were alone when I suddenly heard a husky whisper, "Thelma; I think I'm falling in love." My head spun around. There was no one in sight. Silence followed.

Thelma squeezed my hand. I heard the voice again, even softer this time, "Will you marry me?" What is going on here, I wondered. I heard another voice, Thelma was saying, "Yes, I will marry you!"

I suddenly realized that the strange voice I heard was my own. I had just asked Thelma to marry me. And, she had accepted. We stood for a moment in the soft glow of the streetlight.

Earlier in the day, Thelma and I had been with our church group celebrating Memorial Day picnicking at Tilden Park, high up in the Berkeley Hills. The late spring day was beautiful. Infatuated and blinded by a budding love, I saw Thelma in a new light that day. Together we explored the park. She was a good sport as we hiked in some rugged terrain, over rocks covered with underbrush. I felt like Tarzan courting Jane as she bravely got a firm grip on the rope swing and pushed off to reach the other side of the ravine.

Now at the end of the day, we floated the last block of the walk back to Senior Hall. We slipped into the shadows, by the steps leading up to the dormitory entrance to say our good nights and to affirm our new commitment.

Our unofficial dates had become official and were more in number. A few weeks later, on a Saturday afternoon, we walked to nearby Mosswood Park on Mac Arthur Boulevard in Oakland. We sat together on a soft carpet of lawn as I surprised Thelma with an emerald cut diamond engagement ring. As spring moved to summer, we dated, shopped together, continued our activities at the church, and made plans for a November wedding.

Early in July, Mom and Dad arrived in Berkeley with my younger brother, Larry. He was in the Navy and on his way to a new assignment near Oxnard, California. The trip to California afforded the folks an excuse to help the newlyweds,

Larry and Lu, move from Minnesota as well as get a chance to meet their prospective daughter-in- law, Thelma. Mother was pleased. Dad was impressed. Thelma passed the test with flying colors.

Later in the summer, we flew to Los Angeles so I could meet Thelma's parents. Dad Barnes gave his approval for me to marry his daughter, and Mom was relieved to know that I was not just a figment of Thelma's imagination.

September - From Student Nurse to Graduate Nurse

Thelma graduated from the Samuel Merritt School of Nursing in September. She moved from Senior Hall to the Hospital Nursing Facility next door. She was the only tenant. On a crisp fall evening, Thelma invited me to join her for a home-cooked meal. The dinner included baked potatoes, chicken potpie, a salad, and dessert. Once more Thelma had surpassed my expectations. (Now I admit I am not a gourmet food critic, nor did I see the Swanson frozen potpie carton but - you have to understand - I had been eating peanut butter sandwiches and Campbell's soup, heated on my one burner hot plate.)

I completed my tour of duty with the Navy in January 1955 and enrolled in classes at Armstrong College in Berkeley. I was fortunate to have a part-time job with a public accountant which allowed me to get some practical experience in the field of accounting.

After graduation, Thelma stayed on at Merritt Hospital. She worked in the surgery department. In October she moved from the nursing facility to an apartment on 34th Street within a few blocks from the hospital. This apartment later became our newlywed nest. Neither of us owned a car.

Wedding Bells, Tin Cans, and Our Honeymoon Limousine

Thelma's family lived in Northern California, Los Angeles, and San Diego and West Virginia, and my family lived in Minnesota. We made the decision to get married in our church in Berkeley so that our mutual friends and the California relatives could readily attend. We also made plans to visit Minnesota later in November to spend some time with my family.

On Saturday, November 3, 1956, we joined hands at the altar of the Central Baptist Church in Berkeley. Thelma carried a white Bible, and bouvardia streamers, topped with a single white orchid. She wore a ballerina length gown made of white satin with a bouffant skirt of net and lace.

I must have been so nervous about forgetting our memorized vows that I cannot remember the details of the service, other than a beautiful adaptation of the song *Because God Made You Mine*, and fumbling for the wedding ring.

Rev. Vandenberg, our pastor, gave us some words of counsel, a prayer of blessing and we exchanged our wedding vows. We were pronounced husband and wife. I was permitted to kiss the bride. With heads held high, smiles as wide as the aisle; we led the wedding party directly to the reception area just off the sanctuary, where we shared our three-tiered wedding cake and ice cold punch with our guests.

A shower of rice followed us as we rushed to our "get away" transportation. I had no idea who or when an "aspiring artist" decorated the car boldly announcing "Just Married." Streamers and tin cans were attached to the rear bumper.

Glenn and Beverly dropped us off at the Greyhound depot in San Francisco, as planned. We boarded a commuter bus, destination Sausalito. The bus was crowded, standing room only. We were the only people on the bus with luggage. Thelma proudly sported her Orchid Corsage. I was still in my navy blue suit. No one offered us a seat, so I turned the suitcase on end for Thelma to sit on. As I looked into my bride's dancing brown eyes, I hardly noticed the jostling of the bus or the tired, impatient commuters.

Fifty years later, when we shared this story at our 50th wedding anniversary celebration, Thelma's eyes still danced as we looked back on that day when we turned our sturdy Samsonite suitcase on end. Thelma then had the prominent seat in our "honeymoon limousine."

1956 November – From Honeymoon Bliss – to Building a Marriage

Our three-day honeymoon ended all too quickly. We saved cab fare by lugging our bags down the winding steps from the Alta Mira Hotel to the bus stop. Hungry and penniless we boarded the Greyhound bus for our trip back to Oakland and our waiting apartment.

Because of a short flight of stairs, our first-floor apartment was above street level, a nice feature as it gave us a view of the activity on 34th Street on one side and Telegraph

Avenue on the other. We paid thirty-five dollars a month for our large three-room apartment. The rent included utilities.

Thelma was an only child. I was second born in a family of eight children. For years I had been able to negotiate with my parents and siblings to get my way. As a child I had developed a heart murmur and nervous disorder. To attract attention, sympathy, and to get my way I learned the art of manipulating people. I remember lying on the floor and kicking, crying, sobbing. I may even have learned to produce tears. In the ensuing years, I honed these skills, so they are less devious and more effective.

Thelma, like her father, had a mind of her own. The clashing of wills between Thelma and her father reached the point that he anticipated her requests, raised a hand, and said, "Don't even ask."

In any marriage, adjustments must be made to live in harmony. I had met and married my match. Suddenly, Thelma's wants had a way of becoming needs. Thelma needed a piano. We rented one. Thelma needed a TV so she could watch TV while I studied in the evenings. We bought a TV using credit. We also purchased a small dinette table with four chairs that fit perfectly in the breakfast nook portion of our kitchen.

We often shopped, or window shopped on Saturdays. On one occasion as we walked the fourteen blocks from H. C. Capwells at 20th Street to our apartment on 34th street, we passed a florist shop. Thelma saw a crystal-like vase. She suddenly needed a vase. The ones on display in the window were large and expensive. I put my foot down and refused to budge. Thelma pouted. I sulked. Communication was at a standstill for the remaining ten blocks. Years later, I found the perfect vase at a flea market and smugly made the purchase.

Interestingly, Thelma was attracted to my interest in accounting. She was looking for someone to" manage" her money and take care of her income taxes. I often say, tongue in cheek, "I was looking for someone with earning potential."

On Tuesday morning, the day after we returned from our honeymoon Thelma went back to work in the Surgery Department at the hospital. I returned to my classes at Armstrong College. November fifteenth I deposited Thelma's paycheck in our newly opened joint checking account. (Note: Thelma later admitted it was hard to turn her check over to me.) This was an important step in my accounting career. I became Thelma's personal financial manager and tax consultant. Both of us were now on our way to successful professional careers and big dreams for the future.

With food in the cupboard and a roof overhead, we burrowed deeper into our love nest as we plotted and planned for days ahead when I would graduate, become a real accountant, and we could open a joint savings account.

Richard R. Blake

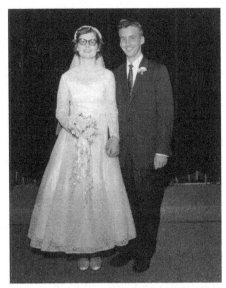

Richard and Thelma November 3, 1956

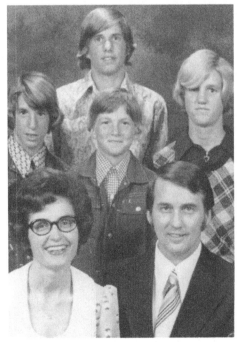

Thelma, Richard, Jim, Rob, Ken, Rick

Combining Family and Careers

Parallel Careers: Motherhood and Nursing

Thelma had dreamed of becoming a nurse as a young child. Her father encouraged her throughout the years that followed. In 1952 her senior year in high school Thelma applied for a scholarship for the nursing program at the Samuel Merritt Hospital in Oakland. The scholarship was granted and in the fall of 1953 she began her training.

By mid-November 1956 Thelma's dream was coming to fruition. Her dedication, positive attitude, curious nature, and deep concern for each patient were recognized not only by her peers, but by the more experienced and seasoned nursing staff and the surgeons as well. These initial traits followed Thelma throughout her 50 years of nursing.

Our first child was due to be born in June of 1958. Thelma, eager to make plans for the baby's arrival resigned her position at the hospital, and traded her operating room scrubs for maternity dresses. She set up a nursery and shopped for baby clothes. The weeks of waiting moved slowly for Thelma as she "played house," cooked for me, and visited with friends over coffee.

Rick was born on June 22 at the Merritt Hospital. Although a patient, Thelma entered into the exhilaration of the trauma and crisis going on around her in the hospital ward. The three days in the hospital, customary in 1958, were stimulating and created in Thelma a secret desire to get back to nursing.

Within weeks of Rick's arrival Thelma was back at Merritt Hospital working on the night shift. We arranged with an agency for a woman to come for a few hours each day to care for Rick while Thelma slept. Rick and I slept the hours that Thelma was at the hospital. However, the plan did not allow adequate rest for Thelma. Within a few short weeks Thelma reluctantly resigned and put her nursing career on hold.

In the summer of 1959 we moved from our apartment to Hayward, a fast growing suburb of Oakland. Thelma's father loaned us the money needed for a down payment on a new tract home with five rooms including three small bedrooms. I was able to finance the balance with a GI loan at a low interest rate.

I became a commuter and Thelma became a full time homemaker and mother. We got to know our new neighbors as together we built community fences around comfortably large back yards, where we sowed grass seed anticipating the growth of a lawn.

We soon were deeply involved in the worship and ministry of Huntwood Baptist Church within five minutes of our new home. We became sponsors of the youth group and an integral part of the congregation.

Kenneth our second son was born on February 9, 1960. Another stay at Samuel Merritt Hospital and Thelma was again homesick for nursing. Kaiser Hospital had recently opened a clinic on the second floor of Grant's Variety store in downtown Hayward. Thelma applied for a position and was soon happily returning to the next stage of her nursing career working part time assisting the surgeon with minor emergencies at the clinic.

My daily routine took on a new complexity. Each morning I loaded playpen, diaper bag, and other paraphernalia into the trunk of the car to drop the boys off at a babysitters on my commute to work. I had to start early since it was a twenty mile drive in rush hour traffic to Balaam Brothers Welding Supply in Emeryville where I worked as office manager/accountant.

Before we were married Thelma and I had discussed an ideal family size. We concluded we wanted a large family, so it was no surprise that in the spring of 1961 Thelma was wearing maternity clothes again. Thelma's nursing career was back on hold.

Our third son, Jim, was born September 13, 1961. Shortly after Jim's arrival Florence Nightingale tapped Thelma on the shoulder again. She answered the nudge by applying for a night position at nearby St. Rose Hospital. Thelma was ready to go to work when the results of her employment physical came back. Test results revealed that Thelma was anemic. Night duty was out of the question. The role of being a mother won out and Thelma again resumed the task of homemaking and the joy of motherhood.

The neighborhood on Aragon Avenue in Hayward was made up of other young couples buying their first homes and starting families. Thelma and the boys all made friends easily. Time passed quickly. In 1963 Rick started kindergarten at Ruus School on Tennyson Avenue. We were still very involved at church.

Ministry and Supporting a Family

During that time Thelma and I continued our contact with Glenn Morrison, Director of Youth for Christ, and his wife. We were still actively involved in the Youth for Christ ministry in Oakland. Glenn had founded a para church organization, Follow Up Supply Line. This organization was designed to provide basic Bible study materials to other organizations, churches, mission groups, and individuals.

As a child, I had committed myself to a career in Christian ministry at a summer camp. At the age of twelve, I had little or no concept of what this might entail. But in 1963 I still had a "tugging" that made me want to step out in faith and become involved in "fulltime" Christian ministry.

May 1, 1963 I took that step and became the office manager of Follow Up ministries on a part-time basis as well as office manager for the Greater East Bay Youth for Christ. Glenn was director of both organizations, and the two shared an office on Fourteenth Avenue in Oakland.

During the months that followed, I became very involved in the work and enjoyed the opportunity to fulfill in part a long life dream. As a family, we were growing. Our expenses had increased. The workload at Youth For Christ had risen to the place where they hired someone full time. I continued my work with Follow Up Supply Line and supplemented our income with a part-time job with an increased pay rate at Best Concrete Steps.

Although not an avid reader at the time. I was a regular drop-in browser at Dearborn's Christian Bookstore in

Hayward. I applied there and got an additional part-time job at the book store, a couple of evenings a week and on Saturday. My platter was full.

New Home on Cowell Street

Whether by chance or by plan another visit from the stork was imminent, it became obvious our little start up house was going to be overcrowded. We had enjoyed our home on Aragon Avenue in Hayward for five years as Ricky moved from babyhood to kindergarten. Two of our sons were born during that time; Kenny in February, the year after we moved in, and Jimmy in September the following year. Now ready for a new baby, due in January 1965 we felt we needed a larger home. We began looking in earnest and found a house on Cowell Street in San Leandro. The builder was willing to take the equity in our Aragon house as a trade in lieu of a down payment. We made the move November 1, 1964.

We were excited about our new larger home. Our furniture was sparse but we had lots of room for growth. We now had a four-bedroom house with a large family room, two and one half baths, a large open kitchen with a spacious living room. We were suddenly paupers with a large house but very happy.

Bicycle Accident

Our friends and former neighbors Ken and Diane Remmert volunteered to keep the kids during the move. I dropped the boys off early in the morning before the moving van arrived.

Our furniture was quickly loaded into the moving van by expert movers. We loaded additional small loose things into our car.

Just as the truck pulled away from the front of the house, the phone rang. Kenny had fallen off the back of Donnie Remmert's bike onto the street. He landed on the back of his head and was being taken by ambulance to Fairmont Hospital in San Leandro.

We grabbed the few remaining boxes, stuffed them into our one and only family car, locked up the house and were on our way.

We took Mission Boulevard through Hayward, got on the MacArthur freeway, and took the first exit at Carolyn Avenue and made our way up the hill to Cowell Street. Thelma dropped me off to meet the movers and drove herself to Fairmont Hospital Emergency Department. Fortunately the hospital was only blocks away.

As the truck was unloaded I showed the movers where to put each piece of furniture. The boxes were dropped off in the kitchen and garage. I went about the work putting things in place in a daze not knowing what was going on with Kenny, Thelma, and the emergency room doctors. The telephone did not get connected until later in the day.

I busied myself with unpacking, box after box. I hung clothes in the new closets, put dishes in the new cupboards, and food in the refrigerator. Things began to look organized. At noon Thelma came to report and to see how I was doing. Kenny had suffered a concussion. He was being transferred to Eden Hospital for observation. He would be kept overnight. As soon as Thelma had delivered the news she left me once more to sit with Kenny as long as necessary.

I felt like the new "house" was becoming our new "home" as I emptied boxes, filled the shelves and put the furniture in place. At around eight that evening I greeted Thelma as she returned from the hospital red eyed and exhausted.

She said Kenny was doing fine. The nurses were observing his sleep pattern and awakening him every hour to be sure he didn't slip into a coma. He was to be released from the hospital by noon the next day. She tumbled into bed and hardly noticed all my hard work.

As I dropped off to sleep a little later, I vividly remembered another move in Kenny's life. The four and one half years since Kenny was born had gone quickly as he progressed from the bassinet to the crib, from creeping to taking that first step, and from the high chair to the kitchen table for meals.

In preparation for Jimmy's arrival in September of 1961 we moved Kenny from his nursery crib to a junior bed in a room to be shared with Ricky. This became a traumatic experience for all of us. Kenny reverted from a self-confident toddler to a sobbing "baby," tugging at his "blankie," asking for his pacifier and trying to climb back into the now empty crib. Kenny did not like change.

Now I wondered *how he would feel when he awoke from his concussion to discover he had been deserted by his family, left behind on moving day, did he think he was being left in an institution for adoption?*

I didn't have long to wait before I found out. The loud ringing of our newly installed telephone jarred me from a deep sleep. I jumped from bed to race for the phone. As I picked up the receiver, I glanced at the clock. It was six a.m.

Dr. Close, our pediatrician was on the line. "I think Thelma had better come and get Kenny," he urged. "I was doing early morning rounds at Eden Hospital. Kenny was awake. When he saw me, a familiar face, he grabbed my arm and has not let go since. He will be better off at home with his family than here at the hospital."

I roused Thelma, explained the situation, and within minutes she dressed and was out the door on her way to Eden Hospital to relieve Dr. Close of his unexpected role of guardian. By eight a.m. we were having our first family reunion in our new home on Cowell Street in San Leandro.

Christmas that year was memorable. We had a white artificial tree trimmed with red balls; a moving spotlight highlighted the tree. The tree and the piano were the only items in the living room. Thelma's Cousin Gerald Pearce visited us just before Christmas and presented us with a beautiful andiron set for our fireplace which added a warm feeling to the almost empty room.

Career Changes and a New Arrival

It soon became apparent that the job at Best Concrete Steps was a mistake. Mid-January, I put out feelers to make a change. I realized that I now had three sons, and a wife to support and another baby due to arrive.

An opportunity opened up for me at the Vita Pakt Juice company in Oakland. This change was the first in a series of career steps that led to some good opportunities in the years that followed.

On January 20, 1965, at the very time President Lyndon Johnson was giving his inaugural address, our youngest son, Robert Kevin, was born. I had watched the entire inaugural address as I waited for the announcement of his birth. The newscasters were giving their impressions and summaries, when the door to the waiting room opened and in stepped Dr. Hayden. "Congratulations, Mr. Blake, you have new son, the baby is doing well," he announced.

Because of a small complication, Thelma was kept over an extra day. I think it was this extra twenty-four hour day that determined the next twenty-four years of our life. The call to nursing again became irresistible.

Vita-Pakt

January 22, 1965, I reported in at the Vita-Pakt office, met the staff, and settled into my desk, just in time to leave at eleven to pick up Thelma and Robert at the hospital. I was given the balance of the day off.

That evening, as I watched more reports on Johnson's role as president. I thought about his challenges as he started four years of heavy responsibilities in his job. I left the significant cares of the country and the world to him. I thought about my own responsibilities: our new home, our new son and my new job. I realized that for the Christian each day is an opportunity for full-time Christian service. I went to bed at peace, thankful for all the blessings that had been bestowed upon me and upon our family.

Several steps had taken place in my career to bring me to this point at Vita-Pakt. I had completed seven years with Balaam Brother Welding Supply where I had learned the basic accounting principles; keeping a set of books, being audited annually, and becoming a part of a working team.

Our living room and kitchen had picture windows which gave us a clear view of Castro Valley below us and the hills across the valley. Eden Hospital held a predominant place in the view from our windows. Thelma looked out over the hills and found herself again and again drawn to the hospital site.

Our wall telephone was just left of the kitchen window within easy reach of the table. Thelma could resist no longer. She reached for the phone, dialed Eden Hospital, and asked for the director of nursing. After a short telephone interview Thelma was invited to complete an application, although I like to think she was hired on the spot.

Thelma soon became the manager of the emergency department of the hospital. This was the beginning of twenty-four years of work at Eden Hospital. We continued to share in the role of parenting our four boys, as I became part time Mr. Mom, and Thelma became part time Florence Nightingale.

My Role as Mr. Mom

The boys were all in the kitchen: Rick age eight, Ken age seven, Jim age four, and baby Robert in his infant seat, age three months. Thelma was at work. It was a Saturday. I was striving to get into my role as the perfect Mr. Mom. There were eggshells on the counter, mixing bowls scattered. The cake was ready to pop in the oven. Cake batter on their faces, the boys each had a spoon cleaning out the bowls.

The doorbell rang. I wiped the flour and cake dough from my hands on Thelma's frilly apron and headed for the door. "I'm Don Driver from the Hastings Business School." Salesman Don announced. "You mailed in a request for information about our advanced correspondence course."

A bowl crashed to the floor. Baby Robert, frightened by the deafening crashing sound, begin to cry. The boys ran for cover. I scowled at the salesman. His foot was in the door. He opened his briefcase. "Why didn't you call first?" I almost shouted, my blood pressure escalating. "Can't you see I can't talk now?" I tried this time to control my voice. Brochures in hand, he smiled.

"You sent in the card!" Salesman Don reminded me as I ushered him out the door. I quieted Robert, popped the cake in the oven, picked up the broken bowl, took off the wilted apron, and wondered how I could resign my position as Mr. Mom.

When Thelma was working the evening shift at the hospital, I usually tried to have the boys in bed by 8 o'clock so I could have a couple hours to myself to relax. Daylight savings time threatened to change this. The boys were instructed to be in the house when the street lights went on; which had not yet caught up with daylight savings time.

One evening after I settled our boys in bed, the neighborhood kids were playing right outside our front bedroom windows. One of the kids, Lisa Tellus, was in our driveway below the window calling out to the boys in their bedroom. The boys rushed to the window to answer her call. I stormed out of the house, grabbed Lisa by the arm, marched her across the street, and rang the doorbell. By the time her mother, Marie, answered the door my heart was pounding, my breath short. I relinquished Lisa to her mother, hardly able to articulate my frustration, turned on my heel and left. Although Marie was speechless and looked flabbergasted, amazingly she somehow understood my predicament.

As the boys grew older, we made arrangements for them to spend a few weeks each summer with my parents and my siblings in Minnesota. We entrusted the boys to the airlines, boarded them on the plane, and crossed the San Mateo Bridge to the peace and quiet of our temporary "empty nest."

Eventually my role as Mr. Mom changed to just being Dad to four great sons.

Careers and Christian Ministry

Medical Team in Mexico

Earlier chapters have told of our Christian heritage, and our mutual desire to be active in sharing our faith personally with others. We did this through our continued involvement in Youth for Christ, and our participation in a local church ministry.

While doing some "research" for our story, I reread a copy of a Bay Area Youth for Christ newsletter from 1954 that highlighted Thelma's involvement in the YFC program. She served as a counselor, assisting in the office and participating in a Bible Study Class. Thelma was quoted as saying, "As student nurse I am planning on using these skills in a mission outreach program."

Four years later my story was featured in our Bay Area Tractor Company newsletter. The article mentioned that my goal of becoming a missionary had been put on hold, and how these goals could be accomplished within the secular setting.

Book Stores

In 1975 my mother came to California to take care of our boys while we went to South America. We went first to Quito, Ecuador where we visited friends at HCJB, Christian radio station. My sister, Edna Headland, and her husband, Paul, met us in Quito and we traveled to Colombia with them to see their work with Wycliffe Bible Translators.

When we returned from our trip we shared the highlights of our experiences with Mom . She told of the adventures of the boys. Mom also expressed an unfulfilled dream. She would have liked to have a combination, book, card, and gift shop with a Christian emphasis.

Shortly after Mom had returned home I noted a "For Rent" sign on a store window in San Lorenzo on my way to work at Bay Area Tractor. I thought about Mom and her dream.

I began to dream her dream with a bit of a selfish twist. Maybe I could entice Mom and Dad to move to California if she would partner with me in a bookstore venture. Thelma and I were regular browsers at the thrift stores and a local flea market. I had already assembled quite a library of used Christian Books, as well as a collection of favorite mystery authors.

Soon Mom's dream became my obsession. I rented the vacant store site in San Lorenzo with the idea of being on a part time basis until the folks could arrange to join us in California. They never took the opportunity; however, that small beginning changed my plans for the next 30 years. Within three years we opened a second store and an outlet at our home church, Redwood Chapel in Castro Valley. I was fulfilling my dream of having a self-supporting Christian ministry.

The first opportunity for fulfilling Thelma's "mission calling" came in October 1977. She joined a medical team of doctors and nurses, sponsored by the Christian Medical Association. Thelma loved serving along with the others in the "Angel of Guadalupe Clinic" in the Guadalupe Valley of Mexico. She came back bubbling with excitement.

Exchange Students

About this same time, we were introduced to the Youth for Understanding program sponsoring exchange students from all over the world. Over the next three years we hosted Luiz from Brazil, Hugo from Argentina, and Anders from Sweden. Each of these boys shared in our family activities for six months to a year while attending our local high school. They joined us on Sunday mornings for services at our church.

The students understood very little English when they came. Our boys were exposed to the Spanish, Portuguese, and Swedish languages and cultures.

In later years we hosted students from Japan visiting Canada and the United States through the Pacific American Cultural Exchange. These students attended English classes at our church during the morning, had guided tours sponsored by the program in the afternoon, and shared family time with us the remaining hours of the week and on the week-ends.

One of these students summed up his visit this way, "I had only three weeks, but these three weeks were very full. This summer is the best of my life. I never forget Dick and Thelma. Don't forget me please. And, I'm looking forward to meeting with you next year. So see you then." And he did. He came back on his own the next summer while on a tour of the United States and a short visit to Vancouver, Canada.

Other guests who shared their lives with us include David from Iran, and Kum Wah from Malaysia. Kum Wah is still an active part of our "family" more than twenty five years later. This note was received from him July 4, 2020.

I walked to your former home. I haven't been back to see your house after you guys moved. When I saw it just now, I teared up thinking of a half a decade of precious memories I had with you and Thelma while living and visiting you in this house. Thank you both from the bottom of my heart for being such a gracious and caring American host family, and having me as the 5th son you never had! I would not be in my current situation if not for you guys and your graciousness. Thank you for sharing the gospel with me and leading me to the most precious gift for mankind, Jesus Christ!

Over the next fourteen years, 1994 through 2008, Thelma had the opportunity to minister with teams from Campus Crusade, the Christian Chiropractic Association, and other church groups, in Russia, the Ukraine, Siberia, Romania, and Mexico. She never met a stranger and she radiated love and acceptance of people. Even when she began to decline the teams welcomed her participation on their trips.

Audit for Mexico Branch of SIL

My turn finally came in 2006. I had the opportunity to use my accounting skills in a foreign mission setting.

My role as an internal auditor was to review the onsite accounting records at the Wycliffe (SIL) branch in Mexico City, and those at a Translation Center in the mountains in the southern state of Oaxaca. By 2006 there were translations of the New Testament available in 113 indigenous languages of Mexico. By 2019 that number had climbed to 151. At the center I had the privilege of interacting with some of the translators.

Thelma and I were able to visit the Mayan Ruins on the weekend of our week in Mexico. On Sunday we attended a Spanish speaking church, sang praises, and listened intently to the message and prayers in the Spanish language. I was able to catch a few words that I had picked up in a college course and while tutoring English as a second language to three Mexican brothers working in the San Francisco area.

We spent the second week in Arizona at the headquarters office for the Mexican SIL branch. A volunteer CPA headed our team; I worked closely with her during work days as we completed our report. Thelma was able to minister to a group of women in a Bible study and prayer fellowship.

It was a moving experience to be able to get a glimpse of another culture and to see firsthand Bible Translators in action.

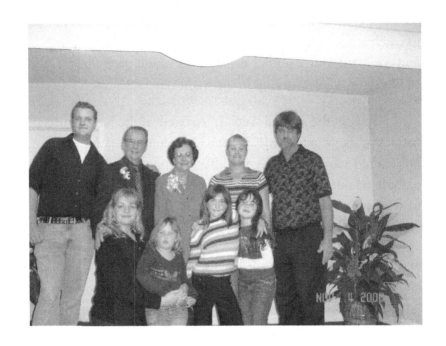

Our Fiftieth Anniversary with Kenneth's Family

Part Two The Seven Stages of Alzheimer's

STAGE 1: NO IMPAIRMENT

DURING THIS STAGE, ALZHEIMER'S IS NOT DETECTABLE AND NO MEMORY PROBLEMS OR OTHER SYMPTOMS OF DEMENTIA ARE EVIDENT.

STAGE 2: VERY MILD DECLINE

THE SENIOR MAY NOTICE MINOR MEMORY PROBLEMS OR LOSE THINGS AROUND THE HOUSE, ALTHOUGH NOT TO THE POINT WHERE THE MEMORY LOSS CAN EASILY BE DISTINGUISHED FROM NORMAL AGE-RELATED MEMORY LOSS. THE PERSON WILL STILL DO WELL ON MEMORY TESTS AND THE DISEASE IS UNLIKELY TO BE DETECTED BY LOVED ONES OR PHYSICIANS.

STAGE 3: MILD DECLINE

AT THIS STAGE, THE FAMILY MEMBERS AND FRIENDS OF THE SENIOR MAY BEGIN TO NOTICE COGNITIVE PROBLEMS. PERFORMANCE ON MEMORY TESTS ARE AFFECTED AND PHYSICIANS WILL BE ABLE TO DETECT IMPAIRED COGNITIVE FUNCTION.

PEOPLE IN STAGE 3 WILL HAVE DIFFICULTY IN MANY AREAS INCLUDING:

- FINDING THE RIGHT WORD DURING CONVERSATIONS
- ORGANIZING AND PLANNING
- REMEMBERING NAMES OF NEW ACQUAINTANCES

PEOPLE WITH STAGE THREE ALZHEIMER'S MAY ALSO FREQUENTLY LOSE PERSONAL POSSESSIONS, INCLUDING VALUABLES.

Stages
1: NO IMPAIRMENT
2: Very Mild Decline
3: Mild Decline

Subtle Changes

Forgetting Meetings at Work

Stage 1 is described in the Part One of the book, Thelma had no detectable symptoms. She was a very efficient nurse functioning at a high level.

By 1994 Thelma and I were enjoying an empty nest. Things were going smoothly at home. I continued doing much of the work around the house as well as all of our personal finances, which had been the normal for us. Because I did so much of this I did not notice any of the memory loss mentioned in Stage 2.

Thelma at age 59 was working as manager of the emergency department at Brookside, a large community hospital in the San Francisco Bay Area. She was in the very early stages of the disease but I did not recognize any perceptive memory issues up to that time. I was not aware of it but Thelma was apparently experiencing a mild cognitive decline that impacted her ability to effectively carry out some of the routine duties, such as the paper work, of her job. She began forgetting meetings and found it increasingly difficult to keep up with the heavy responsibilities of her demanding position.

In addition to managing the emergency department, Thelma was completing the final requirement for a Master's Degree in Nursing Management. She had worked in Nursing Management for many years so the material was familiar to her. The tests were frequently made up of true or false and multiple choice questions, that helped jog her memory. She was able to successfully complete her classes.

Questions for Reflection or Discussion

1. What was happening to Thelma who was still working in a highly responsible position?
2. What signs might Richard have noticed at this early stage that could have made him aware of changes?
3. What were the first signs you noticed that made you concerned about your loved one?

Abrupt Decisions

Although Thelma had finished all her classes for the program, a written comprehensive examination was also required to receive her MA degree. By 1995 she had difficulty focusing on the material. In the past she had easily memorized outlines or lists in preparation for exams but could no longer organize her thoughts to write the detailed answers required in an essay exam. After months of studying she decided not to take the exam and to accept a certificate in lieu of the degree.

I was very disappointed, frustrated, and troubled by Thelma's decision not to take the exam. I still had not realized she was having serious memory issues. Not only did she decide to just accept the certificate, she abruptly resigned from her position in the emergency room at Brookside Hospital. Another decision that left me baffled. Only later did I realize she (we) had begun her (our) journey with Alzheimer's.

For the next four years Thelma worked part time in a less demanding position in Home Nursing. She also helped teach classes in CPR and Advanced Life Support as well as Cardiac Classes for the American Red Cross.

Questions for Reflection or Discussion:

1. What were the abrupt decisions that Thelma made that were indications things were changing?
2. Has your loved one done anything similar?

Forgotten Items

I often overreacted to the small things. I needed to guard against doing that. On Thursday Thelma provided a fruit salad for her Bible Study group luncheon. She left the Tupperware container at the church. In the afternoon, she had an appointment with her hairdresser. She left her umbrella at the shop. Needless to say I was frustrated.

On the following day, on my way home from the gym, I ran some errands, dutifully picked up the Tupperware at the church. We made a "big deal" out of our luncheon date at Home Town Buffet, picked up the umbrella on our way, and capped it off by shopping at Big Lots and the 99 Cent Store. Stuffed and happy by midafternoon, we were at home again and relaxing. We were ready for an evening of reading, television, and a game of Scrabble.

I was worried about what was happening and what the future would hold. I wondered *what will happen next? Will I be able to cope?* At the moment life was still simple and good. We had so many blessings. I needed to be careful about falling into a "pity party" mentality.

In our marriage Thelma and I have worked together at using our strengths and weaknesses in a team effort to support and raise our family. Over the years I may have assumed the dominant role in our home and family life due to various shifts in Thelma's career as a nurse. She had always participated in some of the meal planning and preparation. However, lately it has become necessary for me to take over planning for the evening meal to keep us on a reasonable schedule.

Thelma still enjoys shopping, but often over shops, buying more of what is already on our shelves and omitting priority items on her list. We resolved this by incorporating shopping with our weekly lunch date.

Questions for Reflection or Discussion

1. What little things frustrate you (lost items, over shopping, repeated questions?)
2. How do you recognize the impact on your loved one's ego as they lose independence?

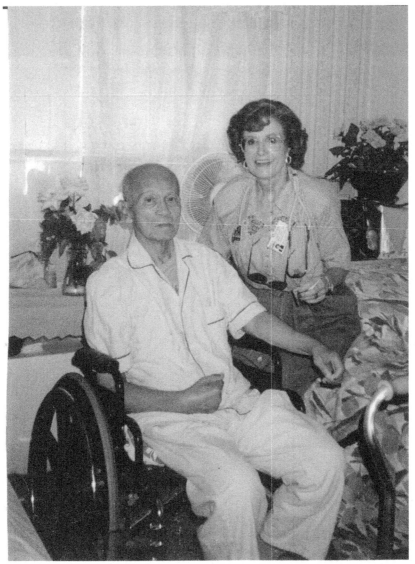

Thelma doing home health care.

STAGE 4: MODERATE DECLINE

IN STAGE FOUR OF ALZHEIMER'S, CLEAR-CUT SYMPTOMS OF THE DISEASE ARE APPARENT. PEOPLE WITH STAGE FOUR OF ALZHEIMER'S:

- HAVE DIFFICULTY WITH SIMPLE ARITHMETIC
- HAVE POOR SHORT-TERM MEMORY (MAY NOT RECALL WHAT THEY ATE FOR BREAKFAST, FOR EXAMPLE)
- INABILITY TO MANAGE FINANCE AND PAY BILLS
- MAY FORGET DETAILS ABOUT THEIR LIFE HISTORIES

Stage 4: Moderate Decline

Caregiving Stress Begins

Wake Up Call

During my annual physical examination in 1999; the doctor got my full attention when – with a sense of alarm and an unusual sternness in his voice he warned, "Dick, your blood pressure is dangerously high." I was given a prescription for lowering my blood pressure, a date for a follow up appointment, and instructions reinforcing the importance of finding ways to lower my stress level. This was a wakeup call. I wasn't even aware of how much stress I was under. That day became a marker in our journey with Alzheimer's.

By this time I was more aware of the reality that Thelma was manifesting additional signs of memory loss. We were also experiencing the added stress of caring for her mother who was in an advanced stage of Alzheimer's. I felt desperate and called the Alzheimer's Association in San Francisco for help and enrolled in one of their classes designed for caregivers.

I learned some important lessons during the four weeks of the class. I became aware of the correlation of the seven stages of Alzheimer's and the impact on a caregiver's health and stress level. Awareness of these stages helped me understand and better prepare for the journey we were facing. I also learned that commitment to caregiving is a family affair, a commitment to communication, of becoming informed of the disease and of making others aware of the disease and of resources available. It was a commitment to Thelma, a commitment to self, and a commitment to watch for the signs and dangers of caregiver burnout.

Thelma was in early stage four of Alzheimer's disease (Moderate Decline). She was forgetful, confused, and feeling anxious; using denial as a defense mechanism. She started to buy memory pills, but never verbally admitted she had dementia. Once she told her sister-in-law whose mother had Alzheimer's, "I pray every day I won't get that disease."

I, too, was experiencing denial, frustration, impatience, and anger. We never discussed together what was happening. I didn't want to think about what was ahead. I also didn't want Thelma to become depressed thinking about our future.

Repeating answers to the same question over and over became exasperating. I tried to create new answers to these repeated questions. Later I learned from an Alzheimer's workshop leader that giving a different answer only further confused Thelma, as she was still trying to grasp the first answer to the question.

Questions for Reflection or Discussion

1. Has your loved one recognized or acknowledged she/he has Alzheimer's?
2. What steps might Richard have taken earlier to better understand the extent of Thelma's dementia status?
3. What was causing Richard frustration?
4. How was the stress of seeing the changes in Thelma affecting Richard?

5. What emotions or frustrations are you facing as a caregiver?
6. How do you as a caregiver deal with your stress?
7. What resources are available in your community that offer assistance to Alzheimer caregivers?

The Missing Oldsmobile

Love is longsuffering.
Love never loses patience.
Love never loses its temper.
Love looks for ways to be kind when abused.

Our Pastor's sermon today was taken from passages from Galatians, Romans, and First Corinthians. I determined *this is good stuff; I can surely put this into practice.*

Ninety minutes later I had my chance. Thelma came to find me in the church bookstore to let me know she was leaving for home. We had arrived in two cars that day, a common practice for us. I told her I would leave in about twenty minutes and meet her at home.

Within minutes she returned. "Dick, I can't find my car," she exclaimed. Ready to react, I remembered the sermon of the morning, sighed, tried to put on patience, and headed for the street in front of the church for a visual check. "I don't remember where I parked," she pondered, "I may have parked in the upper parking lot at North Campus."

We decided I would drive her around the corner to the upper lot to spot her car after I closed the church bookstore.

Meantime the church door had locked behind us. More inner groans, my patience once more being tested we headed around the church to the main lobby entrance.

Later, as we were ready to leave, Thelma decided to get her keys out to have them available when we reached the car. They were not in her purse. After two or three mutual searches, the information desk, the store counter, tables, etc. Thelma checked the lady's room. Finally, we concluded she had left them in the car.

We drove around the corner. The car was not in her usual spot on James Avenue. We did not see it in the upper lot on North Campus or in the main lot.

We circled the route a second time; Thelma logically concluded, "Someone stole my car." By now Thelma was upset and praying for divine intervention. We decided to go home to report the theft. I contemplated how I could explain to the sheriff's office the loss or theft of our car.

Frustrated and desperate, I fought the inclination to harangue Thelma. It's just a car, I thought, Thelma is here with me. Safe: Maybe this lesson in patience would avoid a more severe crisis in the future, an experience with more severe consequences. Someday I will have to intervene and take away another symbol of independence from Thelma, trying so desperately to maintain in her battle for dignity.

As we turned onto Cowell Street, we were relieved and surprised to see Thelma's car in our driveway. We both breathed a sigh of relief. Sheepishly, Thelma remarked, "Oh, now I remember, I couldn't find my keys, and Kum Wah took me to church this morning."

Weeks later I found the keys. On Saturday, the day prior to the missing automobile, we attended a wedding. Thelma transferred a few things from her purse to a much smaller bag. Nestled in the bottom of the bag were the missing keys.

Love is longsuffering.
Love never loses patience.
Love never loses its temper.
Love looks for ways to be kind.

Questions for Reflection or Discussion

1. What lessons have you learned about patience as a caregiver?
2. What is your source of inner strength to meet these challenges?
3. On a scale of one to ten – What is your "endurance" level?
4. When is it time to think about getting a Power of Attorney?

Another Change

In 2004 I closed the San Lorenzo book Store. In late 2005 we decided to sell the San Leandro store I had owned for twenty five years. I put it on the market in October and by December 6th we had a contract for the sale of the building.

We had 30 days until closing! In that thirty days I had sales with greatly reduced prices on everything in the store, gave books to other Christian stores, packed up the rest and moved it to our garage.

In the midst of the sorting and packing the executive pastor of our church came by the store. He told me of an job opportunity in the church business office and asked if I would be available. I said I was. I agreed to start the part time job at the church on the Monday, after the FUMI staff conference.

Questions for Reflection or Discussion:

1. What were the advantages of Richard selling the bookstores at this stage of their journey with Alzheimer's?
2. Have you or do you need to make this type of change in your life at the stage you are at?

Keeping a Flickering Romance Burning
Journal Entry January 16, 2006

It is surprising how I appreciate coming home each day after a five-hour workday three days each week. Maybe the morning trips to the gym and my part time job overseeing the accounting at the church on a regular basis help me deal with the extra stress I face at home in our struggles with Thelma's Alzheimer's.

This week I felt guilt creep in when I agreed with Thelma in some of her confusion. I have the urge to correct her, but Thelma works so hard at communication trying to piece together an incident or, multiple events, with an accurate time line or sequence; my challenging a fact only creates more confusion.

It is difficult for me to see her struggle. It is easier to move on to a table game (even if we flex the rules) or a quick dinner date at Denny's.

Friday we went to the Prime Outlet mall in Tracy for few hours. The forty-five minute drive each way made it seem like real date. It made Thelma feel special. I try to be creative to find small ways to make something happen each day to please her.

Questions for Reflection or Discussion

1. At this time in your journey, what are some small things that bring a brief moment of joy or bring pleasure to your loved one?
2. What are the benefits of a conversation even when your loved one can not remember words or put thoughts together?
3. Are there activities, games, or projects that you and your loved one have enjoyed in the past that you can still enjoy?
4. How do these activities deepen your feelings toward your loved one?

Richard R. Blake

Guilt and Frustration
Journal Entry January 23, 2006

Several days last week were hard as I was making plans
to attend the annual weekend retreat for the Follow Up
Ministries International (FUMI) board members and staff. I
had decided it would be best if Thelma didn't attend, due to
the tight schedule and my active involvement in the program.

We had discussed this many times during the last few
weeks, and Thelma seemed okay with the idea; until last
Thursday when she realized it was coming up Friday. She
tried to put a guilt trip on me. I sometimes made plans without
communicating with Thelma at a pace she could grasp. This
time I thought I had communicated clearly and that she had
understood. I felt badly but I held my ground and did not
acquiesce.

A friend came to the rescue by making plans to take
Thelma shopping and out to dinner on Friday night. Thelma
did fine on Saturday, knowing I would be home in the early
evening.

The bunk bed at the retreat site was hard, so I got broken
sleep. I kept wondering how Thelma was doing and feeling a
twinge of guilt over leaving her. Despite lack of sleep
Saturday went well and plans were put in place for the
upcoming year. Although the schedule was tight, the staff and
board had an opportunity for close fellowship and
camaraderie. I knew I had made the right decision leaving
Thelma behind, and what a welcome home I received.

Questions for Reflection or Discussion

1. What made Richard lose sleep and feel guilty when he was on the staff retreat?
2. Do you have difficultly communicating plans with your loved one?
3. How have you been able to solve the problem?

Does Trouble Really Come in Threes?

One afternoon Thelma was driving down Foothill, on her way home. The red light, at the intersection of Foothill and B Street in Hayward, turned green. As the long line of cars began to move Thelma eased her foot off the brake and the car began a slow roll forward. The car ahead had not moved, Thelma gently put her foot on the brake, she felt a slight nudge from the car behind.

Within seconds the young driver from the car behind Thelma jumped out, camera in hand shooting pictures of an invisible scratch on his bumper, supposedly the result of an impact.

"Are you alright? Are you hurt?" Thelma asked with concern in her voice.

Like a masseuse massaging an aching muscle the young man was tenderly rubbing the unseen spot on the bumper of his car. Traffic backed up, drivers impatiently watched the scene as Thelma and the young man exchanged phone number and addresses, Thelma was relieved that the young man was not hurt. When the light changed to green both drivers eased back into traffic.

That evening Thelma related her experience to me. I examined her car, no damage. The incident was soon forgotten, but not for long.

The engraved return address on the envelope read, J. Milford Mulholland, Esq., Attorney at Law. Belatedly we called our insurance agent, filled out an accident report and again returned to routine. Attorney J. Milford Mulholland seemed determined to alter our agenda. On behalf of his client the attorney filed a claim with our insurance company.

On a Sunday morning late in October, a second incident dramatically changed our timetable. Thelma had been sick in the night with stomach cramps and nausea.

I was in the kitchen having breakfast when Thelma called me from the bathroom. "Dick I need your help." Sensing urgency in her voice, I rushed to her.

"I can't get up," she said. Together we got her to a standing position. Suddenly I felt the dead weight of her body pulling me down as she slumped back to the floor.

I ran to the phone, dialed 911. I reported our emergency. "Is she breathing?" the operator asked. "I don't know, I'll check." I replied. I returned to Thelma, conscious now and breathing. "Don't move," I ordered. "I'm talking to 911.

Somehow I got Thelma back in bed. The fire department arrived first. The hubbub of the next few minutes is now a blur. The walls of our bedroom closed in on me. Two fireman, two paramedics, their oxygen tanks, a gurney, and other paraphernalia filled the room. Within minutes the team had Thelma strapped on the gurney, in the ambulance, and on their way to the Eden Hospital emergency department.

Still in my robe I explained to the concerned, curious, gawking neighbors what had happened. I then quickly dressed and headed for the hospital.

The medical team had already administered a medication to ease the discomfort and were hovering over Thelma in the examining room.

The doctor concluded Thelma was dehydrated from heavy vomiting and diarrhea. He attributed the problem to possible food poisoning from a highly seasoned taco salad consumed on Friday, two days earlier.

Suddenly Thelma became agitated. The medication caused a severe allergic reaction. Full attention now focused on counteracting the damage. Edgy and jumpy, Thelma begged to go home. I was left to try to calm her as the two medications interacted.

The emergency department team continued to monitor Thelma. Midafternoon our regular physician came by. Thelma again pressed the issue of going home. Dr. Chin expressed concern. "Thelma, you come by the office tomorrow if you are not feeling better."

Late that afternoon a nurse and I helped Thelma from a wheel chair to the car. I took Thelma home. She slept the remainder of the evening and throughout the night.

Monday morning I reported for work as usual. At lunchtime I went home to check on Thelma. She was weak, very weak. It was obvious she needed to visit Dr. Chin's office. Half walking, half dragging, we got to the car. I checked out a wheel chair at the medical building and took Thelma to Dr. Chin's third floor office.

After one glimpse of Thelma's pale color and slumped form propped in the wheelchair, the nurse whisked Thelma into an examining room. She rushed from the room for additional help and to make arrangements for immediate admission to Eden Hospital.

Test results revealed that Thelma was bleeding internally from a stomach ulcer. Blood transfusions were started immediately.

On Tuesday I received two calls, one from Kaiser Hospital. Thelma's mother was in the emergency department being treated for pneumonia. The second call came from a State Farm Insurance adjuster asking for a deposition from Thelma regarding the claim filed by Attorney at Law, J. Milford Mulholland, Esq.

State Farm decided to contest the claim. The deposition was postponed, but it was essential that I take Thelma's car to an auto repair shop in Hayward for damage repair estimates and photographs. An appointment was made for Wednesday morning.

Wednesday morning, after checking in at my office, I visited Thelma at Eden Hospital, kept my appointment at the State Farm garage, transported Thelma's mother from Kaiser Emergency to a convalescent hospital nearby and returned to a very pale Thelma at Eden. She was receiving her sixth unit of blood.

More tests concurred with the diagnosis that Thelma was bleeding from a stomach ulcer. Along with the blood transfusions, prescription drugs, a positive attitude and the prayers of family and friends soon put color back in Thelma's cheeks. By the end of the week she was released from the hospital, returned home and was on the road to recovery. The problem with the ulcer never recurred.

I breathed another sigh of relief when Thelma's mother was released from the convalescent hospital and returned to her Alzheimer's residence care home. Life was returning to normal. However, we still needed closure in the unresolved car insurance claim. In the weeks that followed Thelma gave her deposition statement.

A series of phone calls and correspondence followed. The insurance company was standing their ground, as was J. Milford Mullholland. We were caught in the middle. I was well on my way to developing my own ulcer.

Early one evening in late November, a process server presented us with papers. We were summoned to appear in small claims court in Hayward. A representative from State

Farm Insurance Company assured us we had nothing to worry about. If for some reason we lost the case, the insurance company would pay the claim and the court costs. Nevertheless we still felt pressure. In small claims court the plaintiffs and the defendants must represent themselves. Attorneys and insurance agents (as in our case) may be present but they cannot speak for their clients.

We were well coached by the insurance representative of the court procedure. She planned to meet us in the courtroom for moral support; however, her schedule would not allow her to be present for the entire hearing. Thelma became anxious and concerned about relating her side of the story. We entered the courtroom just before 2:00 p.m. as summoned. The courtroom filled up quite quickly. There were several cases scheduled for the afternoon as well as a case carried over from the morning's docket.

The judge entered the courtroom. We all stood. I took a second look. I thought for a moment I was on television in the courtroom of Judge Judy. I looked for the cameras. None were apparent. As individuals presented the claims and counter claims this lady judge mixed common sense, sarcasm, humor, legal terminology, and the wisdom of Solomon in her decisions.

After many years of watching the Perry Mason television series as well as the reruns I was enjoying the courtroom experience. I felt a combination of curiosity and empathy for the participants as the dramas unfolded. It was five-thirty when our case was finally announced.

Thelma and I stepped forward.

The judge opened our case file as she listened and followed along as the claimant summarized his argument. He was suing for chiropractic bills for treatment he said were a result of the accident. I was nervous for Thelma as she told her story of the incident. She told of being a nurse and of being concerned for the young man's welfare. She told of the camera so readily available for pictures of damage she could not see. I was allowed to tell of the findings of the insurance company. Insurance inspectors had visited the complainant's home to take pictures of the alleged damage. The judge reviewed the complete report the insurance company had submitted.

Statistical studies provided by the insurance company indicated that the impact of the car would be like a fall from a chair to the floor. The judge pointedly asked the claimant, "Young man, why are you suing this lady?"

He faltered as he replied, "Well, Your Honor, when I was in high school, I was in an accident and this attorney got a good settlement for me, so I contacted him again." I could hardly believe my ears. Visitors in the courtroom snickered.

The disapproval of the judge was obvious to all. By now it was after six o'clock. The judge sighed as she closed the file and informed the young man that the results of her decision would be mailed within the next ten days.

We watched the judge as she left the courtroom visibly shaking her head. A few days later, much to our relief, we received the court's decision. The judge had ruled in our favor.

Both Thelma and her mother were recovering. We had won our day in court. Thanksgiving and Christmas were just around the corner. We had a lot of catching up to do.

Questions for Reflection or Discussion

1. What are some markers you have faced in your Alzheimer's journey?
2. What steps do you think Richard should take at this stage of his journey with Thelma?
   Regarding: Confidence in Thelma's Driving Skills?
3. Is it time for Richard to get Thelma's medical power of Attorney and other papers in order with a lawyer?
4. Are your loved one's papers in order?

2008 Year of Decisions

Resigned Part Time Job

My health continued to be affected by our journey with Alzheimer's. In addition to the high blood pressure diagnosed earlier, a blood test in the spring of 2008 confirmed that I had Type 2 diabetes. I resigned from my part-time employment at Redwood Chapel to become Thelma's full time caregiver at the end of September.

On my last day of my employment the staff surprised me with a farewell luncheon. They shared some beautiful tributes of my years on the team. Thelma beamed as staff members shared their stories of working with me. I was experiencing a deep appreciation of the Christian fellowship and camaraderie of "family."

After that nice send off, I came home to the reality I would be at home 24/7. I would no longer be with other staff in the church office. I would be home with just Thelma. I wouldn't be tending to the finances of the church. I would be home doing laundry, getting meals, and tending to Thelma.

Thelma gradually declined. Her dementia issues continued to worsen.

Questions for Reflection or Discussion

1. How was the stress of caregiving affecting Richard's own health?
2. What was the first big decision Richard made in 2008?
3. How is caregiving affecting your health?

4. What decisions are you facing at this time in your journey?

Our First 911 Call – Fall of 2008

Thelma had a standing hair appointment every Thursday afternoon at 1 p.m. We had recently made a change to a beautician closer to home. The shop was in one of the many storefronts on East 14th Street in San Leandro. Although the route was direct, the driveway entrance to customer parking at the rear of the building was easy to miss.

Confident that Thelma could find her way home, we had established a pattern of taking two cars. Thelma would follow in her car as I drove ahead leading her into the driveway to the parking lot at the rear of the building. Once Thelma was safely in the shop, I would return home.

One beautiful sunny fall day, we were ready to leave for her hair appointment when Thelma stubbornly snapped, "Dick, I don't need your help. I know where I'm going."

Rather than face her obstinacy, I yielded to her wishes and with misgivings let her go alone.

About thirty minutes later I received a call from the beautician casually asking if Thelma had forgotten her appointment.

I panicked – explained the problem and rushed to the shop. Thelma must have missed the driveway and driven right past. I stood in front of the shop watching traffic both ways hoping to spot Thelma's car. The attempt was futile. I returned home to await her homecoming.

An hour passed. I called 911 to report my concern and was referred to the Alameda County Sheriff's department. Within a short time two officers came to the house to get additional background information to open their file. As the officers were getting the make of car, the license, and other helpful information the front door opened. Thelma casually walked in.

I blurted out, "Where have you been?"

"I was out driving," she innocently replied.

She neither questioned the sheriff's car in the driveway nor the two officers in our living room.

The officer's closed their file, suggested that I make sure she had identification papers with her at all times, and bid us a "good day."

Thelma was happy to be home. She had no awareness of the seriousness of the situation. I was relieved for her safety.

Unfortunately, I did not take any further action at this time. It took several other incidents for me to acknowledge that it was no longer wise for Thelma to be driving. In retrospect, I could have avoided a lot of frustration, conflict, and stress by taking immediate steps to ensure that a safety plan was in place.

Second Call to 911

About two months later, Thelma had a dinner date with a close family friend, Wanda Lorber; a once-a-week treat for both of them. Sometimes Wanda came to our home for a short visit before they went to Denny's Restaurant near our house for an early evening meal.

On other occasions, Thelma visited Wanda for the afternoon before going out for an early dinner. The drive to Wanda's entailed a complicated route through Hayward. Thelma had made this trip often, maneuvering through a maze of complex dead ends, courts, and through several streets to arrive at Wanda's home. I was fully aware of their plan and gave no thought that anything might go wrong.

I had my dinner, did some reading, and enjoyed a couple hours relaxing. As the sun was setting around seven forty-five, I began checking my watch from time to time, anticipating Thelma's return. When Thelma hadn't returned by 9 p.m., I decided to call Wanda. In response to my question, "Is Thelma coming home soon?"

Wanda sounded alarmed, "Dick, she left here two hours ago."

Now I was alarmed! But I tried to sound logical and confident as I responded to Wanda. (I thought I knew the ropes, this being my second 911 call.) "I'll call 911 and ask the police to put out an alert to watch for the car."

I nervously dialed 911 and reported Thelma's absence, gave them the license number. I waited fearing Thelma had been in an accident.

Within a few minutes, two officers from the Sheriff's department were at the door. I invited them in to explain Thelma's evening itinerary and the fact that she had not yet come home from her dinner with a friend as well as the information I had gotten from Wanda.

The lead investigator opened his notebook. I thought he seemed skeptical of my account of her absence. With pen poised, he began to ask questions: the description of the car, the license number, and then – he looked me right in the eye – and asked, "Is there a reason she might not have wanted to come home?" "Did you have a fight, ah, a misunderstanding?"

As though right on cue, the phone rang. "Dick, I'm lost, I don't know where I am." Thelma was able to tell me she was at a convenience store on Mission Boulevard. She got the address from the store manager. One of the officers immediately volunteered to pick her up. We made arrangements for him to lead Thelma home.

Thelma must have made a right turn instead of a left on Mission. She had been driving around for the last two hours. I breathed a sigh of relief, tried to relax, and readied myself for an interrogation.

However, as the other officer and I patiently waited, the conversation took on a note of understanding as I related to him a little of the dilemma with Thelma's dementia and the fine line of personal dignity and the reality of the disease.

An hour later, Thelma was quietly resting at my side. As I offered up a prayer of thanksgiving for her safety. I realized the time had come. She had to give up driving!

Throughout the next few days, I tried to convey this to Thelma. She fought the idea tooth and nail. I succumbed once more to Thelma's determination.

Questions for Reflection or Discussion

1. Why didn't Richard act to put a safety plan in place after Thelma's first incident?
2. How can you avoid the same problem?
3. Has your loved one been lost? How did you handle it?
4. Has your loved one had to give up driving? If so how has that decision affected him/her and you?

Neglecting Self Care

Thelma's nursing instinct continued to manifest itself in concerns for aging friends. On one occasion during this period Thelma was visiting a friend at the Sunbridge Health Care facility in San Leandro. Thelma's friend had recently broken her ankle and was recuperating and receiving therapy for her injury. For the third time in a ten-day period I was sitting in the lobby of the facility while Thelma spent time with her friend.

The lobby and front desk area was crowded with patients, their visitors, and a busy staff. Patients with walkers and in wheelchairs longingly edging toward the main door of the facility, were waiting for family members or perhaps an opportunity to escape. I was relaxed reading a book in an overstuffed chair nearby.

I frequently glanced up to study my surroundings, noting the caring attention the health care workers gave to the wandering patients, often redirecting their attention and the direction of the path of their walkers.

Growing old gracefully is an art, and I'm not an artist, but as I waited for Thelma in the lobby that day I could see the confused state of many of the patients. The stage of my own caregiving experience made me very aware of the fragile balance and amazing capabilities of our minds.

I smiled at nearby patients with my crooked half-smile hoping I was coming across as sensitive and warm.

Suddenly, I became very aware of my unshaven face when I realized that well-meaning visitors were giving me that same "Hello. How are you?" greeting and smile they were giving the patients. The stress of caregiving was taking it's toll.

Questions for Reflection or Discussion

1. How was caregiving affecting Richard's personal care and health?
2. What are you doing to take care of yourself?
3. Who is available to help you have the time you need for respite and personal care?

Decision to Move

In the early summer of 2008 we took our usual month-long vacation at a rental a cottage in Bethany Beach within easy walking distance to Rick's house.

In addition to the barbeques on the beach of Lake Michigan, weekend sightseeing trips, and family times with Rick or Rob, I was subconsciously envisioning life in Southwest Michigan.

On this visit, we explored a new housing development in Stevensville within five minutes of Rick's home. One evening as we visited with the boys we were discussing the possibility of making a move to Michigan. Casually one of the boys asked, "Mom, what do you think?" Her response surprised us all! "Well, if Dick is going to move, I guess I'll have to move with him."

In other years Thelma had vetoed even a hint of this kind of talk. I hid my excitement but was already making plans for the transition.

When we got back to California we asked Jim how he would feel if we moved. He said, "Dad, go!" We had finally made the difficult decision to leave the congested streets, busy freeways, and high cost of living in the San Francisco Bay area and move across the country to a small town in Michigan.

We hired a contractor to complete some needed repairs, upgrades, and maintenance in preparation for selling the house.

Between routine appointments and church activities in the months that followed we sorted, packed, and decided which of our many keepsakes, and accumulated "stuff" we would have to leave behind. Every two or three weeks the truck from our local thrift store came by to pick up the items in boxes and bags set out in our driveway.

Questions for Reflection or Discussion:

1. What made Richard decide they should move across country?
2. Are you considering a move? What factors do you need to consider?

Car Totaled

I decided it was time for us to sell Thelma's car. Earlier in the year, just as Thelma was backing out of her parking spot at a busy Castro Valley Shopping area, a teenage driver in a large pick-up truck rammed into Thelma. The impact of his vehicle pushed the car back against a light pole. Our car now had damage to both front and rear bumpers.

No one was hurt. The damage looked minor. The teenage boy was driving with a learner's permit. The boy's mother and Thelma decided since it appeared to be a no-fault accident, there was no need to report the accident.

Later, when we took the car in for a repair estimate, we found the cost would be more than the Blue Book Value. The car was considered "totaled." We worked out an arrangement for a reduced quote for repairs and went ahead with the work.

However, this required getting the car reregistered with the DMV, and our registration now stated a resale value at $237.00. Thelma was happy to have her car and continued driving.

As we made plans to move to Michigan, I determined we were not taking our cars. I made arrangements to sell Thelma's to a friend for $200.00. His daughter was thrilled with her first car. But Thelma was not happy! She was distraught. She was upset enough about selling the car but was highly indignant at the reduced price.

Questions for Reflection or Discussion

1. What made Richard decide to sell Thelma's car?
2. Have you had incidents like this with your loved one?
3. Why was Thelma upset about selling the car?

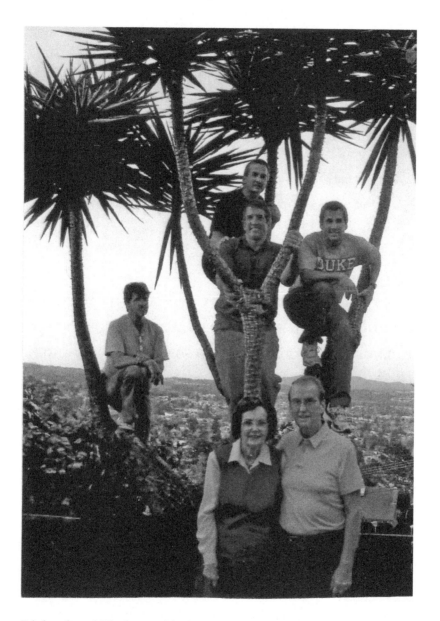

Richard and Thelma with their sons, Ken Jim Rick Robert saying "Good Bye" to the home where they grew up.

STAGE 5: MODERATELY SEVERE DECLINE

DURING THE FIFTH STAGE OF ALZHEIMER'S, PEOPLE BEGIN TO NEED HELP WITH MANY DAY-TO-DAY ACTIVITIES. PEOPLE IN STAGE FIVE OF THE DISEASE MAY EXPERIENCE:

- DIFFICULTY DRESSING APPROPRIATELY
- INABILITY TO RECALL SIMPLE DETAILS ABOUT THEMSELVES SUCH AS THEIR OWN PHONE NUMBER
- SIGNIFICANT CONFUSION

ON THE OTHER HAND, PEOPLE IN STAGE FIVE MAINTAIN FUNCTIONALITY. THEY TYPICALLY CAN STILL BATHE AND TOILET INDEPENDENTLY. THEY ALSO USUALLY STILL KNOW THEIR FAMILY MEMBERS AND SOME DETAIL ABOUT THEIR PERSONAL HISTORIES, ESPECIALLY THEIR CHILDHOOD AND YOUTH.

Stage 5: Moderately Severe Decline

Slowing the Pace

Day of the Move

May 9, 2009 became another significant marker in our journey. As we locked the door of our Cowell Street home of over 40 years, a kaleidoscope of memories crowded for my attention.

We had already said tearful goodbyes to our son, Ken, his daughters Jocelyn and Mary and their children, as well as our son, Jim's wife, Irma, our friends from church and the community. Jim had our luggage in the trunk, our cat in the backseat, and we were ready for the ride to the San Francisco airport. Thelma was already looking forward, with the excitement of youth on a new adventure, eager to be in Michigan for Rick's birthday in June.

I was quiet and reflective remembering: our first Christmas, babysitters, and kindergarten classes, little league games, McDonald hamburgers, Thelma's job at Eden Hospital, picnics at Mt. Diablo, Redwood Chapel Boy's Brigade, fifth grade Sunday School, baptisms, foreign exchange students, high school graduations, family Christmas's with the grandchildren, Ken's pigeons, and Rob's dog Buck. I had other memories: the Family Book Center, my jobs in accounting with Balaam Brothers, Boise Cascade, Follow Up Ministries, and Redwood Chapel. One by one of our boys had left home to begin new lives. We had been alone in our home for 15 years. We were in a new stage of life.

Transition to Rural Life

Over the years while visiting our sons, Rick and Rob in southwest Michigan, I had frequently explored the city of Bridgman, while Thelma had her hair done. I was highly impressed with the public library and the Woodland Shores Baptist Church facility.

In the fall of 2008, when we began the process of getting our California home ready to put on the market in preparation for relocating closer to our Michigan sons. We regularly looked on computer websites for homes for sale in the general area near Rob and Rick.

Rick and Holly visited a home in Bridgman that had just reduced the price significantly. Unknowingly, it was the very house I had been looking at on my computer. They liked it and I loved what I saw in the pictures. We made an offer and a down payment with an April 30, 2009 closing date.

We arrived in Michigan on Saturday, May 10. Our furniture was scheduled to arrive on Monday. We spent the weekend with Rick and family and attended Sawyer Highland Church on Sunday. Jeff Dryden, a friend of Rick's since junior high, was now the pastor of the church.

Even though I enjoyed the church in Sawyer, I had a firm conviction that I wanted to become a part of a church in the community where we lived. When I knew we were moving to Bridgman, I visited the Woodland Shores Church website and contacted the pastor of the church, Rev. John Bedford. He responded and sent information on the church.

On Monday morning our furniture arrived as anticipated. By early afternoon our furniture was all in place and box after box was clearly marked and neatly stacked in the garage. The unpacking process began. The remainder of the week our boys or members of their families dropped in to check on us or help with getting us organized.

Thelma and I shopped at the corner market nearby and had dinner or lunch at one of the family restaurants in Bridgman. We anticipated Sunday, eager to visit the Woodland Shores church.

I thought we would be arriving at the church early for a 9:30 service only to discover we were a couple minutes late for a 9:15 starting time. The ushers greeted us at the door and led us down the middle aisle to the third row from the front of the church, on display for all the congregants as 400 curious, and few questioning eyes turned our way, two visitors were coming late and walking to the front.

Immediately after the benediction, Pastor Bedford stepped down from the platform and welcomed us to the church. He invited us to join the coffee time in the new Family Center.

A lady from the pew in front of us gave us a warm welcome. While the lady spoke to us, Thelma made it clear to me that she wanted to go to the restroom. She didn't like other women talking to me.

As Thelma came out of the restroom and we began to find our way to the coffee, a tiny white-haired lady greeted us with a friendly smile and a welcoming handshake. I was impressed by the friendliness of the lady. Thelma, however, hurried on hardly greeting her. We followed the crowd and found our way to the Family Center and the coffee. As people meandered by with their family or friends, they made us feel welcome.

Someone invited us to an Adult Bible Fellowship (ABF) class. It was a class for senior adults ages 50 and older taught by an associate pastor. I found the class stimulating. I chose not to disclose anything about Thelma's unique challenges at that time.

Later in the afternoon we received a call from a man from the church. He offered to take us on a little tour of Bridgman including an ice cream sundae at the Dairy Queen. (Incidentally, we had filled out a visitor's card at the church.)

We discovered our tour guide, Dr. Dale Smith, and his wife, Bobbie, were charter members of the church. He gave us a brief history of the church, pointed out homes of members, and gave us insight into the area. He mentioned places of interest Thelma and I might enjoy visiting at another time.

Thelma quietly enjoyed her ice cream, the social exchange, and the chance to meet new people. I was already confident that Woodland Shores would become our new church home.

Questions for Reflection or Discussion

1. Have you considered a move to be nearer your children or to an area with less traffic and congestion? What are the pro's and con's?
2. What made Thelma uncomfortable when greeted by the two women at church? Why was she more comfortable with the Smiths in the evening?
3. Is your loved one jealous of attention you give to women/men?

Men's Prayer Breakfast

I noticed in the church bulletin that on Saturday mornings there was a men's prayer breakfast at a local restaurant and began to make plans to attend. I had no idea of the trauma this would create for Thelma.

The evening before the scheduled breakfast, I told Thelma my plans for the next morning; she didn't seem to make much of it – not until we were in bed ready for a night's rest. For the next two hours, she cajoled, wept, and talked, then started again. I thought, *It is such a simple thing. I will be home by the time we usually start our day.* By midnight, exhausted, I fell asleep. I hadn't realized how insecure Thelma felt since our move. She didn't want me to leave her alone for even a minute.

In the morning Thelma was still sleeping when I was ready to go out the door. I gently leaned over, kissed her on the cheek, and whispered I would be home in an hour. I left a note on the table letting her know where I would be and when I would return.

The men's prayer group only met a few more times before a break for summer. Thelma accepted the fact that I would be home before she was ready to start her day. However, in the days and weeks that followed, Thelma rarely let me out of her sight. She followed me from room to room in the house. Our lives revolved around each other 24/7.

Questions for Reflection or Discussion:

1. Why did Thelma make such an issue about Richard going to Men's Group?
2. Has your loved one had similar reactions to being left alone?
3. Was Dick insensitive to Thelma's insecurity? What should he have done?
4. How do you balance your needs with those of your loved one's in similar situations?

Adapting to a New Community

Although the Sunday School Classes for adults and the weekly Bible studies discontinued for the summer a monthly small group (Agape Groups) did not disband. We were included in all of the activities of the group led by Pastor Winn Decker. There were six other couples in our group. In June we picnicked at a park by Lake Michigan, in July at the home of the Priebs, and in August at the Lack County

Township Park. Thelma and I were readily accepted as part of the Woodland Shores family.

Another similarity between our church in California and Woodland Shores was the sponsoring of foreign missions. A week in August was devoted to a mission's emphasis. We met in homes to become acquainted with the work of one of the participating missionaries. We attended a meeting featuring a medical missionary in the mountainous terrain of a Muslim country unfriendly to American missionaries. Thelma was immediately drawn into each story the missionary shared.

When the fall program resumed we were pleased to find a Wednesday night supper at the church similar to what we had experienced at Redwood Chapel. We attended a prayer group while others were involved in youth activities, Awana, or the music program.

Thelma was invited to join ladies in a weekly Bible study class. A member of the class provided transportation. Thelma was an active and important part of the group for the next few years. I helped her by answering the questions from the study guide which she then copied into her book.

Among those friends we made at church were Carl and Millie Stasinowsky. Millie was also experiencing difficulty with dementia issues. Thelma and Millie quickly bonded. Carl and I became close friends and relied on each other for support.

Shortly after our arrival in Michigan I enrolled in a Caregiver's Class sponsored by the Alzheimer's Association, facilitated by the St. Joseph Area Agency on Aging.

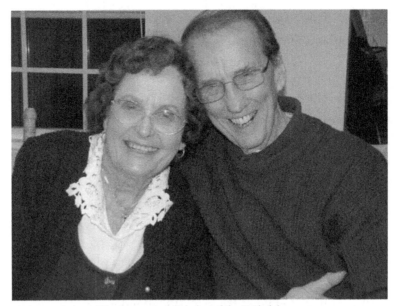

Thelma and Richard in Michigan

Thelma and I both began to adjust to a new life style and liked the change of pace of a smaller community. We enjoyed our new home and the pleasure of being involved with sons Rick and Rob and their families' activities: little league games, family barbeques, picnics, and visits to places of interest.

Questions for Reflection or Discussion:

1. How did Dick and Thelma make new friends after their move when Thelma had moderately severe decline?
2. Have you found it challenging to make friends or keep in contact with friends as your loved one's dementia increases?

Outside Help

In addition to the classroom instruction, Caregiver's Class sponsored by the Alzheimer's Association the agency arranged for respite care for Thelma while I attended the classes. The courses provided help in areas of managing daily life as a caregiver, learning how to get and use help in caregiving tasks, and pointers in taking care of yourself to avoid caregiver's burnout.

We were at that point almost 15 years into our journey with Alzheimer's. Thelma was moving into stage five of the disease; moderately severe cognitive decline. It should be noted the timing of these stages is different for each person suffering from the disease. Thelma focused on past memories and was convinced that her mother and father, both long deceased, lived close by in Bridgman.

One morning at breakfast Thelma asked again about her folks. She accepted the fact more readily they were both gone. That they passed away before we left California and she was there for them when they needed her. However, within an hour she said, "I'd like visit my parents this morning." She repeated that several more times within the next few hours much to my frustration.

I began to realize the magnitude of the disease. Although Thelma was in good physical health, her care continued to become more demanding. She was extremely dependent on me; she wanted to be physically near me at all times.

Carl encouraged me to take advantage of the Adult Day Care provided by Harbor House in St. Joseph. In the summer of 2011, I registered Thelma in the program, for five hours a day, three days a week. Transportation was provided as a part of the service.

Questions for Reflection or Discussion

1. How do you respond when your loved one wants to go visit their relative (long dead), who they are convinced lives right down the street?
2. Have you struggled with the decisions about outside help (either Day Care or Home Health Care) for your loved one?
3. How have you resolved these struggles?
4. What resources are available in your area to help?

Overload
Journal Entry, September 28, 2012

Today was the beginning of week two of Thelma's new prescription, an Exelon patch designed to slow down process of the Alzheimer's disease. It seems that Thelma is showing an increased level of confusion, rather than the expected results.

Yesterday I may have pushed Thelma into "overload." I had difficulty sleeping two nights in a row. As a result I overslept. We skipped our breakfast and usual morning routines to join our senior group at church for a coffee fellowship, which includes hymns, a devotional study, and a short prayer time.

We then hurried off to Thelma's 10:30 appointment in Stevensville for a manicure. We were home by 11:30; had an early lunch. By 12:30 we were on our way to Thelma's next appointment, a permanent at the Kangaroo Klippers in Bridgman. I then returned home, and went back for Thelma at three o'clock.

Once home, Thelma was hungry again. We ate at four instead of our normal five o'clock pattern. As a result we were a full hour ahead of our regular evening routine, which usually consisted of an hour or so of TV, time out while Thelma took her shower, then more TV and 9:30 bedtime for Thelma.

Tired as a result of our full day Thelma exchanged her day clothes for a robe and was sound asleep in her chair by 6:30. I welcomed this reprieve and became deeply engrossed in a writing project I wanted to finish. Thelma slept until around 9 o'clock, awoke rested and wide awake. In a few minutes she got up headed in the direction of the bathroom. I assumed she was going to take her shower; I returned to the computer.

Within five minutes she joined me in the den, smiling, fully dressed, and ready for a new day. More confusion now as I desperately tried to explain it was 9:15 p.m. and bedtime. She conceded and went toward the bedroom. A short time later she returned and asked about eating. I tried to explain about our early dinner. Thelma denied eating anything.

More frustration as I tried to justify my disappointment at Thelma's denial regarding dinner and her growing level of confusion. I then discovered that Thelma had set out a plate of brownies and cheese. Things unresolved and tension building Thelma sat down to eat her small snack.

Again I returned to the computer to finish my project. She soon returned, now dressed for bed. No shower again tonight, something that had started recently but very unlike the Thelma I knew.

Later I crawled into bed, found Thelma's hand, she held mine tightly for a brief moment, whether a reflex action, awake or asleep, I was deeply touched by this sign of Thelma's love for me. Tears welled up in my eyes. The sobs and feeling of helplessness came later in the night. I felt helpless at knowing how to meet all of Thelma's needs and grief over the loss of the perfectly groomed wife I had always appreciated.

Questions for Reflection or Discussion

1. What do you see as the basic reason behind Richard's frustrations?
2. What might have helped reduce the stress level?
3. Who do you see as being in "overload?" Explain why?
4. What lesson or application can you find for this situation from this example?

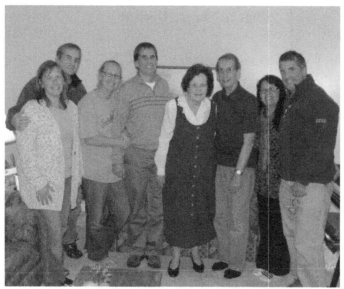

Leslie, Robert, Holly Rick, Thelma, Richard, Irma, Jim

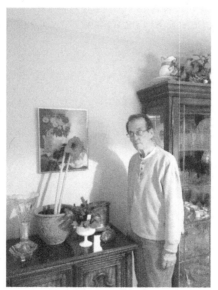

Richard alone at home

Stage 6: Severe Decline

PEOPLE WITH THE SIXTH STAGE OF ALZHEIMER'S NEED CONSTANT SUPERVISION AND FREQUENTLY REQUIRE PROFESSIONAL CARE. SYMPTOMS INCLUDE:

- CONFUSION OR UNAWARENESS OF ENVIRONMENT AND SURROUNDINGS
- INABILITY TO RECOGNIZE FACES EXCEPT FOR THE CLOSEST FRIENDS AND RELATIVES
- INABILITY TO REMEMBER MOST DETAILS OF PERSONAL HISTORY
- LOSS OF BLADDER AND BOWEL CONTROL
- MAJOR PERSONALITY CHANGES AND POTENTIAL BEHAVIOR PROBLEMS
- THE NEED FOR ASSISTANCE WITH ACTIVITIES OF DAILY LIVING SUCH AS TOILETING AND BATHING
- WANDERING

Stage 6: Severe Decline

Painful Decision

Challenges, Frustration and Impatience

By early 2013 it became especially difficult to help with Thelma's bathroom needs. She had always been very private about her personal care and fastidious about her hygiene, make up, clothes, and personal appearance. When she suddenly quit taking her accustomed daily shower, I was desperate. I nervously mentioned this to the staff at Harbor house. We increased her involvement there to 5 days per week and they took over her bathing.

That was a big help but I continued to struggle with frustration, and impatience not knowing how to handle Thelma's increasing personal care challenges. By now I was losing sleep. One night Thelma intentionally or inadvertently locked the bedroom door. I lost my cool as I stood outside the door pounding and demanding that she open the door for me. She seemed to purposely choose to ignore me. My sons became aware of my stress and began to consider possibilities for residential care.

They realized caregiving was taking an increased toll on my health. Over a period of five years a moderate heart valve issue had advanced to severe. I had more tests coming up. If surgery were to become necessary there would be a two to three month recuperation period. Rick questioned me, "Who will take care of Mom if you have to have that surgery?"

I had been concerned for a long time. *If something happened to me how would Thelma be cared for?* I followed up on the suggestion of a friend to explore the possibility of the assisted living care provided by Woodland Terrace in Bridgman. Our family also encouraged me to seriously consider this option. . I appreciated their concern and felt deep down they were right. Still I felt internal conflict *would I be going back on my commitment "for better or for worse?"*

I took the first step. I called and made an appointment with Heather, the director of admissions at Woodland Terrace. On my arrival for the interview a few days later, I met Heather. We chatted for a few minutes, took a tour of the facility, and returned to the conference room in the administration building. I was impressed with the facility, and the well cared for appearance of the residents, the dining areas, and the beautiful layout of well-kept lawns, and other amenities.

Heather explained each of the four units of the facility and the level of care provided in each. I answered a few questions about Thelma and her current abilities and challenges. Together we concluded that Thelma needed the level of care offered in Magnolia Court, the memory care unit. Heather gave me a packet of material explaining the details of the care and policies of Woodland Terrace. She informed me that there were no rooms available in Magnolia. However, we could be put on a waiting list. We would be number three on the list. I had Thelma's name added to the list and continued to pray about the matter.

In early August I had a cardiac catheterization (a test for blockage in the arteries and to determine the condition of the heart value). My arteries were fine but my aortic heart value might have to be replaced.

About the same time I had an upper GI endoscopy. The surgeon took a biopsy. I was diagnosed with Barrett's Esophagus which is a precursor to stomach cancer. Physicians had been monitoring this since the fall of 2009. There had been some change but results proved to be non-cancerous.

Although the test results were encouraging at the time, my health was being affected by caregiving. These conditions would need to be closely monitored. Combining my own health needs and Thelma's increased need for personal care, after much prayer and counsel my sons and I made the decision to place her in Woodland Terrace as soon as a room was available. I was thankful it was readily accessible to our home.

Within three weeks, I received a call from Heather. Thelma had moved up to the number one spot, and there was now a room available. I arranged to see the accommodation and to complete the application papers. I was delighted with the room, located in a quiet corridor yet near the center of group activities. I made the deposit and arranged for Thelma to move in the following week.

Questions for Reflection or Discussion

1. What factors indicate the need for more help in caring for your loved one?

2. How do you decide when it is time to place your loved
   one in a care facility?
3. Have you had disagreements in your family about
   whether to place your loved one in a care facility?
4. How have you resolved those issues?

Resident of Magnolia Court

August 29, 2013 became another marker on our uncertain,
unmapped journey. Thelma became a resident in Magnolia
Court, the secure unit for people needing her level of care at
the Woodland Terrace facility.

I vividly remember that warm sunny afternoon in August.
I sat alone in the car, deeply concerned about Thelma's
transition from the six hours of care at the Harbor House Adult
Day Care Center to becoming a full-time resident at Woodland
Terrace.

I had made arrangements with the Harbor House Adult
Day Care Center to take Thelma to Woodland Terrace at the
end of the day rather than bringing her home. Although I had
discussed the plan with the staffs at both places, I had not
discussed it with Thelma.

I had been alerted by a family member to be prepared.
She had experienced extreme resistance as their loved one
became agitated and refused to cooperate when she was just
going to their home for a few days. To avoid another scene
when she needed to go to a facility for long term care, they
made an appointment with her doctor. He checked her over

and then told her she needed to go to the care facility for a period of time. He had been telling the family for some time he thought she needed the extra care. She was taken in a van right from the doctor's office.

As I sat alone in the car outside Woodland Terrace, waiting for the Harbor House van to arrive with Thelma, I experienced conflicting emotions. I vacillated between guilt and an overwhelming sense of sadness, yet feeling a sense of release as I anticipated relief from the tsunami-like stress that had been escalating over the past few months. I couldn't help but question, *am I doing the right thing?*

I moved from the car to a chair at the entryway of Magnolia Court, the memory unit, where Thelma would be living. From this vantage point I could watch for the arrival of the Harbor House van. I was beginning to feel more apprehensive and guilty as the minutes ticked by. My reverie ended when two Woodland Terrace staff members joined me to meet Thelma. The Harbor House van arrived right on schedule.

A thoroughly confused Thelma stepped off the van. She had no idea of our plans. I introduced Thelma to Heather and Nora, the Woodland Terrace welcoming committee. I explained to Thelma that she would soon be having dinner with new friends at Woodland Terrace.

As our hosts cordially led the way, we entered an open area where residents were gathered together for a late afternoon activity or watching TV. Thelma was introduced to one or two of the staff as the newest resident of Magnolia Court. We went directly to room number 6. By now Thelma was bewildered but compliant. she recognized our familiar small sofa, the blue upholstered rocking chair, the chest of drawers, the family pictures, and her mother's original oil paintings.

Heather and Nora cordially chatted with us, making Thelma feel comfortable in her new surroundings. At just the right moment, Nora asked if she could pray with us. During the prayer Thelma smiled, gripped Nora's hand and appeared to bond with her. Even though I felt assured things were starting off well as our new friends left us, I felt very alone.

We sat on the sofa holding hands quietly lost in our own thoughts. I was at a loss to know how to communicate the reality of the situation. Thelma with a look of uncertainty and bewilderment curiously contemplated the single bed directly across from us. It was the only unfamiliar item of furniture in the room. She looked unsettled, possibly wondering how she and I were going to sleep together in the narrow bed.

As we talked, a friendly staff member came and caringly invited Thelma to join her for dinner. Together they headed for the dining room.

I sat for just a fleeting moment while wet tears streamed down my cheeks. Then I slipped out through a nearby exit with a mixture of guilt and distress. I was faced with my own bewilderment and uncertainty of the next step of our uncharted course of our Alzheimer's journey.

Questions for Reflection or Discussion

1. What did Richard do to avoid conflict both before and at the time of the transfer?
2. What did Richard feel when he left Thelma at Woodland Terrace?
3. Have you been able to talk with your loved one about the possibility of needing residential care?
4. Have you had to put your loved one in residential care? If so what were your feelings?
5. How did the staff make the transfer process easier for both Thelma and Richard?

Alone at Home
Journal Entry September 1, 2013

Today is day number four since we moved Thelma to Woodland Terrace. It has been reassuring to receive excellent feedback from the staff, as well as positive affirmation from Rick and Holly, and a friend from church that we made the right decision. I enjoy watching Thelma show her concern for other residents by trying to help them. She gets involved in some of the group activities and responds positively to the staff.

Alone at home I feel a deep quietness. Thelma is always just below the surface in my thoughts, suddenly appearing in an imagined movement or a sound from somewhere in the house, only to remind me, that she is not here. I am alone. I play soft music in the background to fill the void of being alone.

In the two days following this entry, I prayed, "Father, God, wrap your arms around Thelma today, comfort her; give her your joy and may it be reflected in her countenance."

I continue my prayer. "Help me to trust you today and to rejoice in the knowledge that you are watching over Thelma. Comfort her in her loneliness and confusion. Manifest yourself to her throughout the day."

Questions for Reflection or Discussion:

1. How did Richard feel several days after leaving Thelma in residential care?
2. What did he do to help himself?
3. What feelings have you experienced in a similar situation?

Christmas Party
Journal Entry December 13, 2013

Last evening Woodland Terrace sponsored a Christmas party for all of the residents and their families. Fifteen of us joined Thelma for the Christmas dinner they had prepared for all the residents and their families. There was a spirit of excitement and celebration in the air. Festive decorations, Christmas sweaters, and bright colored clothes added a touch to the gala occasion.

We all gathered around the Christmas tree for a picture with Santa Claus, Mrs. Claus and one of their faithful elves who later delivered toys to Sinai, Kate, Tane, and Lucy. Jack was too small to take part, however note that he's included in the picture.

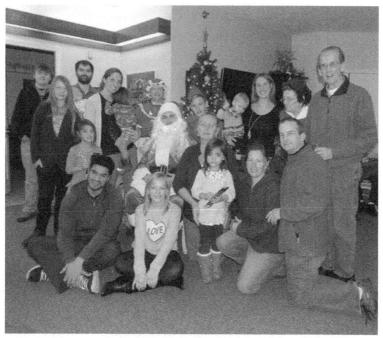

Rick and Rob's families with Thelma and Richard at Magnolia Court Christmas Party

Thelma enjoyed every minute, she seemed to want to stop time, and savor the moments. It is times like this that alert us to the gift of family, the bond of love, and the innocence of children.

We hold on to these moments as we join together to celebrate together the birth of Jesus, our Savior, the promised Messiah, and coming King of kings, and Lord of lords.

Questions for Reflection or Discussion:

1. What made the Christmas party at Woodland Terrace special for Thelma?
2. What have you done or can you do to make the holidays special for your loved one?

Trusting God for the Future
Journal Entry- February 16, 2013

The uncertainty of the future is something that we all face. Jesus admonished us to "Take no thought for tomorrow" and goes on to assure us of God's care. Today as I look out on the a snow covered lawn, I see two small birds feeding and another huddled in a corner on our deck, protected from the wind, fed and protected by a loving, caring, heavenly Father.

This same heavenly Father that cared for Noah and Elijah in the Bible, and is caring for the small birds on my deck has given me a new assurance that He wants me to trust Him for every minute of my future: one minute, one hour, and one day at a time.

Observe and consider the ravens;
for they neither sow nor reap,
they have neither storehouse nor barn;
and [yet] God feeds them.
Of how much more worth are you than the birds?
Luke 12:24

Questions for Reflection or Discussion:

1. Richard found writing his prayers or journaling his feelings an outlet for his pain, frustration and anxious thoughts in concern for Thelma.
2. What do you find helpful for releasing your pain of losing your loved one little by little?

Gratitude for Caregivers
Journal Entry November 9, 2015

I am blessed and I speak for Thelma too.

We rely on a group of individuals, caregivers, whom I have come to think of as friends. These friends provide for Thelma's physical needs with a tender touch, a warm smile, and a genuine sense of sacrificial service and love.

Twenty-four hours a day, seven days each week, they help Thelma through her confusion, comfort her when she is lonely, and tenderly encourage her through her times of edginess, as well as her stubborn moments. They demonstrate compassionate care while monitoring her meals, bathing her, dressing her, making sure her colors don't clash, brushing her hair, applying makeup, and attending to those inevitable "messy" unmentionables. They show their affectionate concern for Thelma's comfort.

These acts of thoughtfulness and kindness do not go unnoticed. The friends I am referring to are the faithful team of caregivers on the Woodland Terrace – Magnolia staff.

There are others we think of as friends of Thelma and friends of Magnolia Court. These are the other residents; some who hover over Thelma in a motherly way, comforting, touching, and affirming; others, as sisters, chatting, laughing, or exasperated, but always loving. There are also the family members of other residents, who, while visiting their loved ones, shower Thelma with smiles, love, and warm acts of kindness.

A core of healthcare professionals, therapists, hospice caregivers, and Woodland Terrace administrative staff, while regularly serving other residents, offer Thelma, a smile, a touch, or a word of encouragement. I treasure each of these deeds of thoughtfulness as acts of love and friendship beyond what I can extend to Thelma. I also benefit from many of these same "friends" as on my daily visits they extend, words of encouragement to me, and express concern for my welfare, both my physical health, and emotional needs.

I am blessed. I am also blessed with a community of friends who demonstrate concern and care. These include our church family, my Alzheimer's support group, the Bridgman "Writer's Group" and the many acquaintances who greet us with smiles and conversation while shopping or eating with friends at nearby restaurants.

And lastly, my family, my four sons, Rick, Ken, Jim and Rob and their precious families; our extended family, those of my brothers and sisters, and their offspring, Thelma's aunts, uncles, and cousins and their offspring. And there is a friend that is closer than a brother; that friend is Jesus. We are truly blessed.

Questions for Reflection or Discussion:

1. Richard expresses gratitude for caregivers and staff and others who relate to Thelma. What benefit do you suppose there is in this exercise?

2. What is your reaction to the staff and others who help with your loved one?

3. Do you have a Health Care Team? Who is your Health care team?

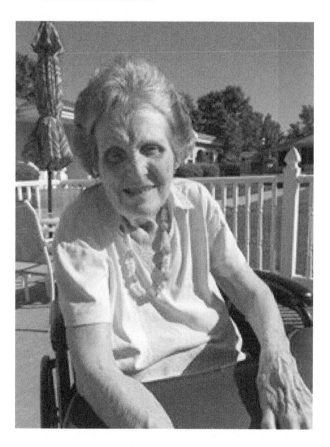

Thelma enjoying the patio at Magnolia Court

STAGE 7: VERY SEVERE DECLINE

STAGE SEVEN IS THE FINAL STAGE OF ALZHEIMER'S. BECAUSE THE DISEASE IS A TERMINAL ILLNESS, PEOPLE IN STAGE SEVEN ARE NEARING DEATH.

IN STAGE SEVEN OF THE DISEASE, PEOPLE LOSE THE ABILITY TO COMMUNICATE OR RESPOND TO THEIR ENVIRONMENT. WHILE THEY MAY STILL BE ABLE TO UTTER WORDS AND PHRASES, THEY HAVE NO INSIGHT INTO THEIR CONDITION AND NEED ASSISTANCE WITH ALL ACTIVITIES OF DAILY LIVING.

IN THE FINAL STAGES OF ALZHEIMER'S, PEOPLE MAY LOSE THEIR ABILITY TO SWALLOW.

Stage 7
Very Severe Decline

Broken Hip, Surgery, Therapy, and Healing

December 2014

December 7 is a day I always associate with Pearl Harbor Day in 1941. Later it became a very significant day for our family as it is my daughter-in-law Holly's birthday.

This day is now etched in my memory as another marker in our journey with Alzheimer's. A telephone call from Woodland Terrace early in the evening alerted me that Thelma had fallen in her room. I was told that she was sitting up in a wheel chair and did not seem to be in pain. Other than the report, there was no apparent concern or any reason for my presence.

The next call came around 9:30 p.m. – urgent this time. As Thelma was being put to bed the charge nurse realized there was sufficient concern for action. Thelma had a possible hip fracture as the result of the fall, an ambulance had been called. I was urged to meet the ambulance which was due to arrive by 10:00 p.m.

I immediately called Rick and Rob asking them to meet me at Woodland Terrace for moral support in what now had escalated to emergency proportions. Within twenty minutes the three of us were at Thelma's bedside awaiting the arrival of the ambulance.

Once the ambulance drivers arrived, things moved
quickly. Thelma was safely secured to the gurney and taken to
the ambulance. We decided that I would ride with Thelma in
the ambulance and Rob would ride with Rick to Bronson
Hospital in Kalamazoo. We were in the ER in the process of
admitting Thelma when Rick and Rob arrived.

By midnight Thelma was settled in her room. Surgery was
scheduled early the next morning. Rick decided to return
home, get a few hours sleep and return in the morning prior to
Thelma's surgery. Robert and I stayed behind for the night's
vigil with Thelma.

Over the next six hours, Robert stayed at Thelma's side,
tenderly making sure she didn't pull out the oxygen tube,
pursuing memories of his EMT training, driving an ambulance
and his frequent trips to Eden Hospital's Emergency
Department where Thelma had been manager.

I dozed a few minutes at a time scrunched up on a padded
window seat a few feet from the bed. Nurses dropped by at
intervals to check on Thelma. They chatted with Robert and
hurried off to other patients. Robert continued his vigil; I
continued in my pattern of broken sleep throughout the night.

By six in the morning the preparation for the changing of
shift began; clatter of breakfast trays in the hall, bright lights
turned on. Thelma's surgery was scheduled for eight o'clock.
Memories of the flurry of pre-op activities are unclear, but I
do remember Thelma's surgery was rescheduled for later in
the morning due to an emergency call for the doctor in charge.

Rick returned as planned. We waited; the rest of the morning is all a haze now.

Transfer to Westwood of Bridgman for Therapy

Thelma responded well to the in hospital therapy. The day came to transfer her to a rehabilitation facility for further therapy. We chose Westwood of Bridgman, near our home and our local family physician.

I rode along as a passenger in the ambulance as we returned to Bridgman. It was dinnertime at Westwood when we arrived. The admission process completed. I arranged with Rick to take me home; exhausted.

Thelma soon found a spot near the nurses' station, I'm quite sure she imagined herself as "in charge" as she watched with wide-eyed excitement, her face lit up. I joined Thelma around ten each morning for a visit when the residents were enjoying coffee and refreshments in the cafeteria just before the daily exercise routine.

Thelma did not progress in therapy as expected. Before the end of the month she was returned to her room at Woodland Terrace.

Questions for Reflection or Discussion

1. What precipitated Thelma's move to stage 7 or Very Severe Decline in her journey with Alzheimer's?
2. Has your loved one experienced a similar incident?

3. How did it affect them?
4. How did your loved one respond to therapy?

December 2015

Letters from Thelma to her Granddaughters

Dear Jada and Ella,

Some of my memories are stored away deep in the memory banks of my brain, but I wanted to pass along to you a couple of things that will remind you of the days when you visited our home both in California and in Bridgman.

Grandpa Dick helped me remember why these tokens of love were chosen especially for you.

Jada, as our oldest grandchild, I wanted you to have something from our wedding gifts. (November 3, 1956). The "Fostoria" dish was given to us by the housemother of my dormitory all through my nurse's training. The dish will remind you of how proud I have been of your choice to become a nurse and the sweet bond of love and respect you have always shown me.

The serving tray seems to fit in with your giftedness in hospitality and entertaining, following in your mom's example. This dish may have come from Aunt Mae or my mother, Nellie Imogene Oldfield Barnes, or from Grandpa Dick's knowledge of my love for beautiful glassware.

Every year while we had the Family Book Center in San Leandro, Grandpa Dick gave me the new seasonal Precious Moments creation. Over the years we have given away nearly our entire collection. This one is special because of the meaning behind it as it relates to Jesus, the Lamb of God, and the reason behind Christmas.

Love, Grandma Thelma and Grandpa Dick, Christmas 2015

P. S. Although I put these words on paper for Grandma, I know she would have liked to express them herself.

Dear Chelsey and Girls,

For some reason, none of us can understand why; I can no longer express my thoughts through written or oral words. Many memories are locked away someplace in the depth of my brain. The exciting thing is that I can still sense the love of family and friends, and I treasured those days when you came to see us while Grandpa Dick and Semisi worked on English as a Second Language and you and the kids watched movies with me…and just loved on me. That same love and caring spirit come through as we watch you demonstrate this gift caring for your friends, family, and one another. The intricate design of the delicate pink candy dish and serving plate seem to suit you, Chelsey, and express your warmth, grace, and a deep sense of God's love.

The little snow boy catching the fresh snow in his face was a gift from a very special friend at our church in

California and reminds me of my junior high and high school years and our snowy winters in the higher elevation of McArthur, California. I hope you will treasure these together with your gift for building memories over the years ahead.

Love from Grandma Thelma (written by Grandpa Dick)

Dear Shannin and Lucy,

Shannin, I want you to have this uniquely crafted book to let you know how I treasure the way you have always displayed faith. You have accepted life's challenges, and moved forward with purpose. I have prayed for you since you were a babe in your mother's arms.

I cheered you on as I watched you on the soccer field, always determined. I listened intensely as you played the piano, intuitively introducing new ways to reach the low notes, in ways no piano teacher would have thought of.

When you came back from your Youth With a Mission overseas' assignment, I listened with interest as you excitedly told of about sharing God's love. Our conversations centered on the Lord Jesus, on our mutual concern for world missions, and our love for music.

You are facing new challenges every day. The other gift I am giving you is a small trivet wall hanging, a reminder that "Faith makes all things possible. Love makes all things easy. And Hope makes all things work.

Love to you and your precious family,

Grandma Thelma (Written by Grandpa Dick)

Questions for Reflection or Discussion:

1. Why do you suppose Richard wrote these letters (from Thelma) and gave special mementos to his granddaughters?
2. What can you do to help your children and grandchildren / nieces etc. have respect and positive memories of their grandmother/aunt?

Transitions
Journal Entry September 16. 2016

Transitions: Even though times of transition are tough, the riches of refinement is worth the pain of loneliness and frustration. Susannah Ince

We are in a new period of transition in our journey as we face the challenges of Thelma's Alzheimer's disease. She is now confined to a wheelchair. Her communication is more limited. I am learning to take away at least one little special remembrance, each day as I visit Thelma: her smile, her attempts to join in a song, the sweetness of the brush of her lips on my cheek, the warm touch of her hand as she tightly squeezes mine. I treasure the blessed memories of the past as I tell Thelma stories of family, friends, and those times we enjoyed together. Today Nell Dale's book *French Fries, Ice Cream & Cucumber Sandwiches – A Poetic Memoir of a Journey with Alzheimer's* came to my attention. Nell captures the essence of the roller coaster of emotions faced by the

119

victims and caregivers of those facing the afflictions of Alzheimer's disease.

In brilliant patterns of poetic prose, Nell describes her journey and the havoc brought about by the ominous diagnosis of Alzheimer's disease. Her poem relates the progression of her husband Al's cognitive decline. In vivid word pictures, she tells of how she went through the stages of denial, loneliness, and of experiencing grief as she lived through the slow loss of her loved one living: but "gone."

Her poem *I Should Have Known* describes the fear and confusion of the early signs.

I Should Have Known

When Al started wanting to leave the symphony at
intermission and the opera before the last act,
I should have known.
When Al bought books he never read,
I should have known.
When Al refused to try a new restaurant,
I should have known.
When Al became agitated when I went out in the evening,
I should have known.

What should I have known? That Al was frightened, frightened that he couldn't concentrate for so long a time; frightened to do something new even though he wanted to do it; frightened to be alone.

Nell sums it up with a question and reveals her thoughtful emotion-filled response.

Would I have behaved any differently if I had known that Alzheimer's was beginning its insidious journey, leaving him frightened and confused.

No, I think not. Because I didn't know Al was frightened, I didn't take away Al's dignity but reassured him; I didn't shatter his protective screen, which would only have left him exposed and vulnerable.

I should have known, but I'm glad I didn't.

Nell speaks of Al's unyielding need for complete attention. She shares keen observations on the unexpected, unpredictable and emotionally draining demands on the caregiver. Nell's willingness to become vulnerable by expressing her deepest thoughts and emotions add another level of credibility to her writing.

Her journal entries and poems reveal an amazing spirit of gratitude and a positive attitude in the midst of the various stages of her journey. Throughout the narrative, mutual love and devotion between Nell and Al demonstrate the strength given and received as new challenges are met head-on.

Nell Dale shares insights into her own life as she faces each new challenge of Al's relapse into "childhood." She tells of her faith, her work, her family, and of caring for Al three years in their home. She relates the story of discovering Barton House and of the loving care Al received while a resident.

A fellow traveler with Nell, I am a caregiver in process. I am reminded of the need to maintain a healthy perspective, to avoid burnout by asking for help, and to accept the challenge one step at a time; I hope that our story, Thelma's and mine will be an encouragement to others on their unique journey with their loved one.

Questions for Reflection or Discussion

1. How do you identify with Nell when she asks: Would I have behaved any differently if I had known that Alzheimer's was beginning its insidious journey, leaving Al frightened and confused?
2. What steps are you taking as a caregiver to avoid burnout and maintain a healthy perspective?

Robert's Accident
Journal Entry, October 11, 2016

The amazingly beautiful October afternoon was shattered when I received the news of Robert's accident. Saturday he was working on a Moped. While doing a test run on Kaiser Road, only a short distance from his home, the bike swerved and went off the road. Robert was thrown from the bike directly into a fence post – head on.

A passing motorist witnessed the accident and immediately contacted emergency services. Robert was taken by ambulance to Lakeland Hospital in St. Joseph. Because of the extent of his injuries, he was airlifted to the trauma center at Bronson Hospital in Kalamazoo. That evening physicians performed surgery to relieve the pressure of the swelling on his brain.

When I visited him on Sunday, Robert was heavily sedated and in an induced coma. Seeing him lying there on machines and unresponsive to my voice was heart wrenching, but it was reassuring to know that he was being well cared for by a dedicated staff.

Today as I write, my heart is very heavy for Thelma, for Robert, and for our entire family. Yesterday I tried to explain to Thelma about Robert's accident. I felt very strongly that it was important for me to attempt to communicate this information to Thelma, even though she is in a state of severe cognitive decline. I tried to explain the seriousness of the situation as step by step I softly related my concern for Robert, our youngest son. I don't think Thelma understood the gravity of what I was trying to relate. However, as I continued to visit with Thelma, dear friends from the Woodland Terrace staff, aware of the situation and concerned for our needs, stopped by her room to offer their support.

As I briefly updated these staff members on the details of the accident and Robert's current status, I tried to include Thelma in the conversation, looking directly into her face as though speaking only to her. Knowing of Nora's Christian faith, I asked her to pray. Throughout the prayer Thelma held my hand, strong and steady. My heart was lifted and I truly felt that Thelma understood and was being reassured that the Lord would strengthen us throughout the days ahead.

Earlier this morning, I visited the website Agingcare.com and found this beautiful poem. The words of the poem help me realize the importance of my regular visits to my sweetheart, the love of my life, Thelma.

Do Not Ask Me to Remember
By Owen Darnell

Do not ask me to remember
Don't try to make me understand
Let me rest and know you're with me.
Kiss my cheek and hold my hand.
I'm confused beyond your concept.
I am sad and sick and lost.
All I know is that I need you to be with me at all cost,
Do not lose your patience with me.
Do not scold or curse or cry.
I can't help the way I'm acting,
Can't be different though I try,
Just remember that I need you,
That the best of me is gone,
Please don't fail to stand beside me,
Love me 'til my life is done.

Questions for Reflection or Discussion:

1. How did Richard communicate their son's accident to Thelma?
2. Have you had similar serious situations? How did you communicate?

60 Years of Marriage

Reveling in Attention
Journal Entry November 10, 2016

Today I stopped Thelma's hospice nurse, Holly, to share with her how well Thelma had done on Saturday as we celebrated our 60th wedding anniversary with the family. I was very eager to tell her of Thelma's alertness over the full four hours of activity throughout the afternoon.

Holly had seen photos of the event posted on Facebook. She agreed that Thelma seemed to interact with the family, appreciate the attention, and enjoy the energy, excitement, and joyfulness of the great grandkids.

She went on to relate how when she was with Thelma recently, she had read to her. Thelma loved this extra attention and listened with interest as Holly read. As she was ready to leave, Thelma spoke two words, "Don't Go." Not as an order but as an affirmation of her gratitude. These two words and special nonverbal affirmations – become the memorable moments I hang on to as I make my regular visits to spend time with my precious Thelma.

Anniversary Book
Journal Entry November 11, 2016

Today as I arrived to visit Thelma she was finishing her lunch. She had eaten her fruit and most of her casserole, and was working at finishing her roll. I asked for a half cup of coffee and joined her at the table. I sipped my coffee and broke off a small piece of her cookie for her and one for myself as well. As she ate her cookie, I cleaned up some of the food she had spilled in her lap; then inadvertently I spilled her remaining juice, embarrassed myself, apologized, and escaped to Thelma's room.

Today I talked softly with Thelma as I massaged her shoulders a bit; I got a few smiles from her. Then I showed her the beautiful 60-year anniversary book Rick's wife, Holly, had made. It had family photos taken over our 60 years of marriage. I quietly shared some thoughts about the boys, their families, and pointed out when and where some of the pictures were taken. As we turned to the last page, we saw a picture of the family taken at Woodland Terrace Family Christmas Celebration two years previously. There were 24 of our family standing by the Christmas tree with Santa Claus and Mrs. Claus. Without hesitation Thelma reached out, her eyes focused on one face in the picture as she pointed directly at me, her satisfied smile and the mischievous twinkle in her eyes lit up the room for me, another memorable moment.

Questions for Refection or Discussion:

1. What seemed to make Thelma happy?
2. What makes your loved one happy?

Daily Visits
Journal Entry April 12, 2017

As I entered Magnolia Court, the memory unit at Woodland Terrace, I spotted Thelma, enjoying an audience participation TV program. I greeted Thelma; alert to the sound of her name, she turned my way, greeted me with a mischievous grin, and extended both hands to welcome my anticipated arrival.

After a few words to Thelma, I greeted a few of the other residents before I maneuvered Thelma, in the wheelchair, to her room for our one-on-one getting reacquainted visit.

Thelma was alert, attentive as she listened to my soft flow of conversation, affirmations, and smiles. Although she could no longer form sentences, she made attempts to add to the conversation through unintelligible syllables accentuated with sparkling eyes and heartwarming smiles.

I shared a beautiful card we had received from friends from church. Thelma reached for it and held it tightly in her fist as she pointed to the beautiful flowers with her other hand. She has difficulty grasping and holding cardstock, magazines, or books, however, she makes a genuine effort to be independent in the process. She still enjoys pretty things.

I opened the Promise Jar, from a nearby table, to remove a now familiar, York Mint Patty, a regular part of our visits. Thelma enjoyed a couple of tiny bites. I offered her water, she sipped the water through a straw, savored the sweet chocolate mint and the cool water. I took delight in being together as bite by bite I fed her the rest of the mint.

Today I was eager to read a children's book to Thelma, a story, telling about Samantha's broken leg and her purple body cast. Thelma's eyes brightened as I read about Sammy's arrival at the Emergency department to see the doctor concerning her broken leg. As I pointed out the pictures of

Sammy in the Emergency Room, the nurses, and the doctor, it was as though Thelma was reliving her days as an Emergency Room nurse.

The time passed quickly. All too soon for Thelma, I reminded her we needed to join the other residents for their daily exercise and song activity. She acquiesced, and we joined the other residents as they were assembling for the morning group time activities.

Today I was rested and alert. Our time was a happy time for Thelma with memorable moments for me. A special time for both of us, truly a win-win visit.

Questions for Reflection or Discussion

1. What are the benefits of one sided conversation even when your loved one can no longer form words or put thoughts together?
2. Why do you think that rest is a significant element in making your experience pleasant?
3. How can you plan to make each visit unique and enjoyable for both of you?
4. What are the advantages of spending some one- on-one time (what I like to call "getting reacquainted" time) as well as group opportunities provided by the activities staff to make it a Win/Win time for both of you?

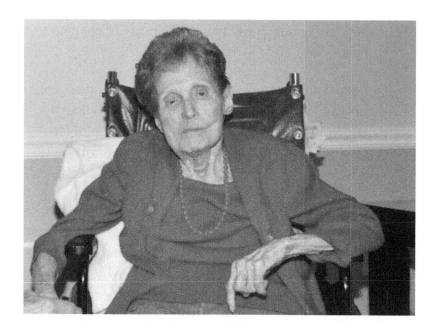

Ambiguous losses
Journal Entry May 13, 2017

Today I actually talked to a bumblebee. Well maybe not a real conversation, I talked. He buzzed. I directed him to the red colored nectar in my humming bird feeder. Never once did I see his wings stop. I wondered if he ever had shortness of breath. He left me to ponder this as the sun peeked out between the clouds in an unpredictable pattern above the trees.

I continued in my reverie as I relaxed in my pre-Father's Day gift, a "glider rocker" stationed on our deck and enjoyed the peacefulness of a back drop of trees that surrounded me

My thoughts turned to Thelma. She is fragile now, less than 100 pounds. She still seems attentive to my gentle words of encouragement, when I softly urge her to share her thoughts with me. Her smile is my reward. Her way of communicating without words, "I do love you, Dick."

In the midst of my loneliness, I sense the quiet gentle whisper of the Heavenly Father, through the cooing of a mourning dove. I look up in awe at the thought of His waiting, too, for me to respond, maybe with a soft smile to acknowledge my love and the awareness of His presence.

The sound of a redwing blackbird at the birdfeeder, calling for his mate, became another reminder of the wonder of God's creation and of His desire for our fellowship. The bumble bee returned, buzzed at me, flew on by, destination unknown. I am now addressing the bee as "honey" as I smile – contentedly alone – but not alone. I continue to remind myself that "Caregiving is Love in Action."

Thelma and I are still sharing the miracle of life, and I want to treasure these remaining days, weeks, months, or years, one day at a time.

It has now been over 18 months since the day I sat at our dining table discussing hospice care services for Thelma. My guest, representing Hospice Care, carefully explained a palliative care plan that would be coordinated with Thelma's present care at the Woodland Terrace facility.

As she stood to leave, she looked out over this same scene; the backdrop of green lawn and gently swaying trees, as though inspired, she softly spoke of the peacefulness and quiet sense of serenity of my home. I needed this reminder as we meet the challenge of a new marker in our journey with Alzheimer's.

Alzheimer's research and independent studies reveal a relationship of pre-death grief in the experience of dementia caregivers. These studies address issues of ambiguous loss, as this relates to the grief process brought on by stress, the burden of caregiving, and the consequent tendency to develop depression. Ambiguous loss happens as a result of seeing the person we once held dear become someone else.

Ambiguous losses include the loss of friends, loss of social life, loss of flexibility, loss of dreams, and the loss of hope.

A positive look at these ambiguous losses have given me new hope, challenged me to be alert for opportunities that will nurture emotional stability, spiritual growth, and creativity.

Questions for Reflection or Discussion

1. Have you found it harder to stay in touch with friends? How has this impacted your sense of loss?
2. How do you meet your social needs? How have you built flexibility into your heavy responsibilities as a caregiver?
3. Did you see yourself in my reverie and observations of the birds and the "honey bee"? Or did you feel, *I think Richard is in serious need of therapy.*
4. How do you keep hope alive in these difficult days of "grief" over ambiguous loss?

Markers along the Way
Journal Entry – October 18, 2017

In December 2013 when Thelma had surgery for a hip replacement we wondered if it might be her last Christmas with us. In 2015 after she entered the Palliative Hospice Care program due to a major weight loss and open sores, we wondered again if she would make it until Christmas. In November 2016 we celebrated our 60th wedding anniversary and then another Christmas.

Now as we face another anniversary and another Christmas, we understand the power of love better. We will stand together to face the next storm that comes our way.

Throughout this emotional roller coaster ride we have been on for the last many years I have been losing my Thelma. My roles become complex: protector, caregiver, and a regular visitor at Woodland Terrace.

As I entered the dining area, I called out, "Thelma." She looked up with a broad grin and a matching glow in her eyes. In recent weeks Thelma has evidenced difficulty with chewing and swallowing her food. As a result of this, she has been put on a soft or pureed diet. I often plan my visits to arrive during her meal-time. The staff monitors her eating with a minimum of help. Thelma likes to be independent in feeding herself. Sometimes she rejects the staff's offer of help. Although I actually get a personal satisfaction out of the process of helping Thelma with her meals, I limit my practice of feeding her to a minimum.

The words Alzheimer's and dementia often bring tears to my eyes as we continue to face an unknown but somewhat predictable future. I have come to recognize that Thelma is reaching the final stages of a progressive disease. Each individual's experience will be different; however, there are certain markers along the way that are similar but vary with each person. Some may have more difficulty with one than another.

1. Inability to perform tasks associated with personal care
2. Incontinence
3. Inability to communicate verbally or through written expression
4. Weight loss
5. Skin breakdown
6. Difficulty chewing and swallowing

Although Thelma has now experienced all of the above symptoms and is confined to a wheelchair she still demonstrates a desire to be independent, enjoys people, and responds well to individual attention.

Thelma continues to surprise us all: our family, the Woodland Terrace staff, and the medical team caring for her, as she bounces back after every hurdle. I still call Thelma my princess, I think of her as my sweetheart, love her as my wife, and cherish her as the mother of my children.

Questions for Reflections or Discussion

1. What symptoms from the list above is your loved one experiencing at this time? Do they have other

symptoms not mentioned on the list? How are you handling it?

2. Are you familiar with "Palliative Hospice Care?" How do you feel about it?

3. What are the advantages and disadvantages of helping with Thelma's meals?

4. How can feeding her become a win/win for all involved?

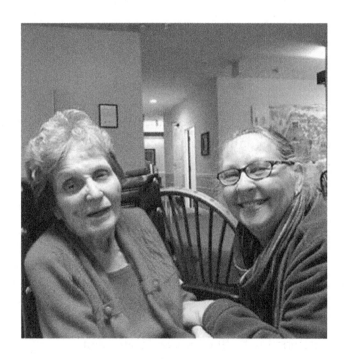

Thelma and Rick's wife Holly at Magnolia Court

Nearing the End of the Journey

Tears
Journal Entry Week of November 5, 2017

Yesterday's impressions, but food for the stars,
lost in the night
Today's new plans take shape, in the theater of hope
On the threshold of tomorrow
Dim awareness, the blessing of sleep
God's master plan of re-creation

On Monday last week, I arrived at Woodland Terrace around 10:00 expecting to see Thelma at her place at the breakfast table. This is one of the days during the week she is scheduled with a team of Hospice Caregivers for a shower. I went to Thelma's room. The door was closed. I knocked, thinking she may be getting dressed. Getting no response I opened the door, entered the room, and to my surprise her wheel chair sat in the middle of the room empty.

A mixture of panic and curiosity raced through my mind as my eyes scanned around the room -- no Thelma! I glanced again at her bed against the wall. There was hardly a wrinkle in the coverlet. Then I saw the form of her slight body, like a small, misplaced decorative pillow under her blanket. Thelma was still asleep. I felt a wave of sorrow realizing how thin and fragile she has become. *Were we nearing the end of our downward journey.*

I deliberately watch her sleeping as I pull up a chair to wait a few minutes before rousing her. I quietly watch as Thelma sleeps, she shifts slightly. I realize she is dreaming, as she utters a familiar "don't," betraying a troubled dream. I hold back tears, biting my lower lip to stifle a sob as I feel the raw emotion of the anticipatory grief of a loving husband.

Today rather than filtering my thoughts through a Pollyanna perfect network of wishful thinking, I allow myself to wallow in the reality and impact of the dread disease of dementia on Thelma's intellect, psyche, and physical reflexes.

Tenderly I say her name, "Thelma, it's Dick, I'm here to see you." She stirs, opens her eyes a bit closes them and seems to sleep again.

I silently wait. I rub her back and whisper "Thelma."

She turns to face me now, eyes open. I read into her smile, "I'm glad you're here."

She reaches out her gnarled hand - her lips don't move, but her eyes plead, "I don't know where we are going, but will you walk with me down this path of uncertainty?"

I nod my head slowly and mumble my tearful commitment to continue our journey together.

Questions for Reflection or Discussion

1. Have you had similar feelings in your experience with anticipatory grief? How do you work through these emotional moments?
2. Do you feel Richard is looking at caregiving realistically or through "rose tinted glasses" of unreality?

Unintelligible attempts to Communicate
Journal Entry November 18, 2017

Thelma makes a sound, an unintelligible attempt to communicate. I smile looking into her eyes. "Tell me what you're thinking," I ask. "Let's talk some more about what your day has been like."

Thelma laughs a combination grin and giggle. Our eyes meet as Thelma smiles in a warm, self-satisfied way. I gently touch her hand.

Her eyes close. I quietly watch Thelma rest, her face relaxed, peaceful, tranquil, and serene. I find paper and pen and begin to write.

Her eyes open briefly. She watches my pen as I scribble words on the page. I tell her, "I'm painting with word pictures, as I create your portrait on my paper. She seems to like this idea. Her face shows a kind of curiosity, love, and acceptance. I have come to understand that our inner feelings do not always have to be expressed vocally. Thelma's eyes and her smile say it all.

I understand it usually takes about two years to work through the stages of grief. It isn't often you can share this grief together with your loved one. Thelma and I are traveling that journey together, one day at a time. But in another sense I am alone as I have faced the ambiguous losses over the years of losing Thelma little by little. Now I am dealing with anticipatory grief as I realize that soon I won't have her at all.

I am learning new lessons all the time as I relinquish Thelma's care more and more into the hands of others while I deal with the apprehension and anxiety that accompany the uncertainty about the future of this journey.

I am getting a better understanding of the truth that God never intended for us to walk alone and that our times are in God's hands. I am learning to be willing to become vulnerable, to respect the feelings of other family members.

I am finding a new peaceful closeness to Thelma as we share quiet moments, allowing our mutual feelings together blossom into a joyful hope. I continue to accept the process of death and the conflicting feelings of loss and the agonizing dread of that day.

I draw strength from our assurance of the promise of the wonderful life awaiting us in heaven in the presence of the Lord Jesus.

Questions for Reflection or Discussion

1. Can you identify with Richard and Thelma's unspoken sense of communication?
2. How are you coping with ambiguous loss and anticipatory grief?

Preserving Dignity
Journal Entry Week of November 19, 2017

In recent months I have had more occasions to visit Thelma at meal-time. This enables me to oversee and help Thelma throughout her meal. It also provides me with an opportunity to become a part of the community of Magnolia Court made up of: other residents, their family members, the Woodland Terrace caregiving team, and amazing volunteers that provide various kinds of assistance and encouragement to the residents and their family members.

Dr. John Dunlap's book "Finding Grace in the Face of Dementia" talks about the importance of dignity and respect for the person with dementia. Dr. Dunlap reminded me that most persons, even in the severe stages of Dementia, "seem to do better when others pay attention to them, demonstrating that they are still social beings."

Over the years of Thelma's progressive decline, I have been very sensitive not to discuss memory or dementia issues in her presence. However, over the last year it seems I have become somewhat insensitive. When I discuss Thelma's eating habits or other health issues with the staff in her presence, she becomes agitated.

Although Thelma is at a stage where she relies on body language, facial expressions, and undecipherable attempts at forming words to communicate, her displeasure with the conversation is obvious. This is particularly true if I relate humorous incidents, either past, or current. I realize, once

139

again, the importance of this principle. I need to respect her dignity. She doesn't like to be ignored while I am conversing with others.

Questions for Reflections or Discussion

1. Do we view people with dementia as whole persons, or does their personhood diminish with their cognitive ability?
2. How can a good and powerful God allow such a tragedy? Is dementia meaningless, and if not, what are God's purposes?
3. What is it like to experience dementia?

Fragile but Unwavering in Spirit
Journal Entry December 4, 2017

I thought she was sleeping as I watched her, eyes closed, and steadily breathing. I had come to spend an hour with Thelma alone before dinner this evening. We were in her room. I read a few pages from a Devotional book. She would open her eyes; smile briefly, and drifted off again.

The hospice team had taken extra care today with Thelma's make up, adding color to her cheeks and had carefully added definition to her eyebrows. They do this for Thelma knowing she appreciates it, and knowing how I try to see in Thelma the same sparkle in her eyes and warm smile that caught my attention the first time our eyes met.

I talked aimlessly hoping to get a reaction from Thelma. Her attention span now lasts only a few minutes at a time. As her responses gradually increased and she smiled more often, I tried to interpret her thoughts. I shared newsy things from my day, interjected reminders of her nursing days, current family activities, and expressions of love. With Thelma's soft hand in mine, as I place a light kiss on her cheek, I catch a mischievous sparkle deeply buried in the dark tunnel of her faded eyes. I detect a giggle forming deep within her ready to restore memories of spontaneity and a reckless young couple very much in love.

Although we think these priceless moments shared together are just for us, this evening as I joined Thelma for a surprise dinner date it became a unique family time. We were surrounded by a busy team of remarkable, friendly, concerned and genuinely loving caregivers, the Woodland Terrace, Magnolia staff.

When friends ask how Thelma is doing, I describe her as fragile but unwavering in her spirit – tenderhearted, and caring.

Questions for Reflection or Discussion

1. What steps can you take when the tedium of caregiving gets overwhelming to continue to experience a heartfelt sense of love?
2. How can you maintain the qualities of love, devotion, and romance of first love?

Loving Touch
Journal Entry December 27, 2017

It felt good to be back on our regular schedule today after the busy Christmas holiday weekend. Thelma was alert as I joined her at the breakfast table. She gave me a big smile. Her smile gave me a sense that she was waiting, expecting to see me.

Thelma was in the process of eating her oatmeal, but willingly allowed me to take "control." Over the next 30 minutes, I talked, she smiled. I spooned her food, she ate. It pleases her and me when she eats all her breakfast, including her Boost and fruit juice.

Breakfast finished, we greeted a few of the other residents as we made our way to Thelma's room. Today I busied myself with packing up some of the Christmas décor, cards and other items that had accumulated over the last few weeks.

Thelma, soon tired of watching all my activity, made it clear that she preferred my undivided attention. I sat beside her, looked directly into her eyes, and massaged her neck and shoulders. She had become the real Thelma now; content, relaxed and smiling.

I looked at this as a small miracle of the power of God in a loving touch, personal attention, and the comfort of a gentle voice.

When it was time for the resident's exercise and music activity, we made our way to the community area, where people were already assembling. We found a place where we could sit together next to Louise.

Thelma and I had met Louise when she moved into the Magnolia Court a few months ago. I always greeted her by name during my daily visits with Thelma. Today she was troubled and disturbed. As I settled Thelma in her place, Louise grabbed my hand. I listened, trying to catch the meaning of her words. "I don't understand these people."

Agitated now, she reached for my arms to emphasize her distress. "They always take my arm, and I never know which one they will take next." I took her hand in mine, and tried to assure her that it was okay. She spoke lower.

I wasn't sure what she was saying. It sounded as though she were asking me to pray. I took both her hands in mine, closed my eyes and quietly begin to pray. I asked the Lord to give Louise a calm peace and the sense of God's presence. As I opened my eyes and released her hands, Louise made the sign of the cross, closed her eyes, relaxed and within minutes was sound asleep. This was another small miracle of the power of a loving touch, personal attention, and the comfort of a gentle voice.

Questions for Reflection or Discussion

1. What small signs are you encouraged by when your loved one unexpectedly responds to your unique gift of love?
2. How can you reach out to other residents and their family members to offer a moment of respite to the other caregivers in your unit, family and staff?

3. Does your facility have a caregivers' support group where you can share experiences and give and receive ideas and encouragement from family of other residents?

Final Days

Good Daddy Journal Entry February 12, 2018

The days and weeks since my last journal entry are fast fading into a blurry haze. However, there are some highlights, some bright spots that brought smiles to Thelma and unforgettable memories to me.

As I was spoon feeding Thelma her morning oatmeal, one of those unique, (what I call "Magnolia Moments") took place. Shirley, Thelma's breakfast partner, watched as I coaxed Thelma, "Open wide."

Suddenly Shirley spoke, "You're a good Daddy." Thelma grinned, her whole face lit up, as though in approval. I was deeply touched. Shirley's comment today triggered other memories going back in time to 1965 when our boys were young.

Shirley's words replayed in my mind as Thelma and I left the breakfast table to spend some time visiting in the comfort and privacy of her room.

Today we took an imaginary trip to the zoo through the book *Five Little Children at the Zoo*. As we joined the children in the book on their walk through the zoo, we met a kangaroo, a dove, a peacock, an elephant, and a cow. We also shopped at the souvenir store. I counted the children in the story, pointed out colors, things of nature, and the wonders of God's creation. Thelma nodded a broad grin, an acknowledgment of her awareness, and enjoyment.

I looked in Thelma's eyes as I talked about our "real" visits to the Oakland Zoo, near San Leandro, California where we raised our boys. Together we went back in time. I became a young daddy again, Thelma an innocent child.

I am treasuring those memories and so many more each time I visit Thelma.

On another day, I remembered Thelma's love for our cat Monique. We were looking at a children's story when a black and white kitty trying to catch a butterfly caught her eye. Momentarily I saw in Thelma's expression a sense of the awe, love, and trust of a young child inspired by God's nature. But then suddenly her picture-perfect look of serenity turned to a troubled brow expressing an undisclosed need. She seemed disturbed and distant in her own thoughts, maybe remembering losing Monique.

Shortly Thelma's smile returns. I think she understands my need for an expression of her love. My eyes water, I stifle a sob, squeeze her hand, and acknowledge her response with my smile and nod of acceptance.

Communication and the ability to carry on a conversation are difficult at every level and spectrum of Alzheimer's disease and impact the caregiver and their loved one.

Questions for Reflection or Discussion:

1. What did Richard do to try and make his visits meaningful?
2. How is your loved one's inability to communicate affecting you?

Thelma's Final Days – February 23 – March 1, 2018

I feel more profoundly within myself Thelma's frustration. I am experiencing cognitive empathy, a deeper awareness of the emotional pain Thelma is going through but cannot verbally express.

A note to family and friends, February 27, 2018

I have been telling Thelma, "When Jesus calls your name, take his hand and follow Him to the room or mansion He has been preparing for you."

Thelma is ready to meet Jesus face to face in the next few days, maybe even today. I spent the night with her.

She is resting well; a wonderful staff, loving caregivers, who have become personal friends during Thelma's four and one half years at Woodland Terrace, are working with Hospice Care to ensure that she is as comfortable as possible.

Questions for Reflection or Discussion:

1. How did Richard try to prepare himself, Thelma and his family for the end of the journey?
2. Are you and your family ready to let your loved one go?
3. Have you made final arrangements for your loved one?

Richard R. Blake

Thursday March 1, 2018 - Thelma's Last Day

My prayer this week was for Thelma to experience a minimum of pain. Most of Monday through Thursday, I was at Thelma's side as she went through a series of evidences that the end was near. However, periodically she would respond, open her eyes, give me a loving smile, look in my eyes and smile again.

Today, Thursday morning March first, was different; the familiar responses no longer came. I continued to sit at her side, hold her hand, talk softly, and in my reverie let the tears come. I had slept the last two nights in a recliner chair beside her bed.

A staff member slipped in quietly to check on Thelma. She adjusted the extra pillows and Thelma's position to make her more comfortable. The aid gave me a guarded word of encouragement. I thought I detected tears in her eyes as she turned to leave the room.

Several members of the night crew stopped by to express their love for Thelma; I sensed a genuine concern for providing me with moral and spiritual support. I moistened Thelma's dry lips with wipes and gave her an occasional drop of water from the tip of a straw. Thelma had lost the ability to swallow food, and there was a risk of choking when sipping water.

In the early afternoon, the boys joined me. Close friends and hospice staff dropped by to express their concern, friendship and love for our family.

148

I decided to take a brief reprieve; to go home to freshen up, get a bite to eat, and a brief rest. Before leaving I took Thelma's hand, kissed her cheek, and whispered my love and assured her I would return in a couple of hours.

Within an hour I had eaten a light dinner and had drifted into light sleep in my recliner when the phone rang. It was Rick calling, "Dad, Mom just peacefully breathed her last breath."

I like to think Thelma wanted to spare me the emotional pain of that moment.

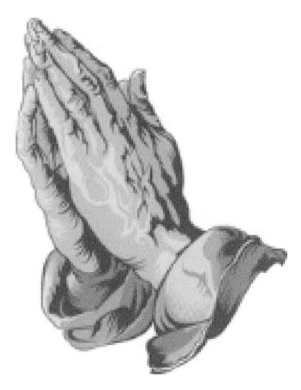

Richard R. Blake

Part Three
Afterwards

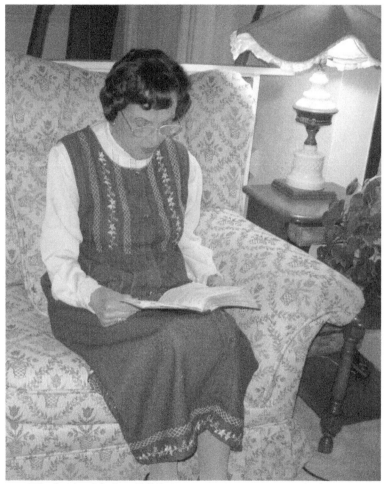

Thelma with her Bible

Celebration of Life

March 12, 2018

The Celebration of Life service for Thelma was held at Woodland Shores Baptist Church. Pastor Jim Oakley officiated. Our four sons were all there: Jim and Kenneth made the trip from California. Rick and Robert's children and grandchildren participated in the service. Ryan Blake accompanied while Elin and Meredith Blake played their instruments to the music of *Be Thou my Vision*, Shannin Vander Ark read Scripture and Sinai Fonua sang *Amazing Grace*. Jada shared the following tribute.

Testimonial by Granddaughter Jada

The words that come to mind when I think of my Grandma are strong, confident, and joyful. She genuinely cared for people in their greatest needs. Physically she cared for others as a nurse. Her love for nursing was evident to all of us and infectious to me.

When I entered nursing school, she was cheering me on, always encouraging my studies, anxious to talk about which classes I was taking. As I got married and started having a family, she continued to encourage me! She was happy as each child was born and laughed with joy every time we visited. But she was always sure to encourage me to keep studying, to keep learning and growing in nursing.

She cared for the physical needs of others, but even more, she cared about their deepest spiritual needs. At the front of her thoughts was sharing the hope of salvation through Jesus Christ. I don't think anything made her happier than a conversation about Jesus. I remember sitting at a baseball game with her and sharing about a Bible study I was in, and her whole face lit up as she asked me to tell her all about it.

She spoke to me with such intimacy and attention, like I was the most important person to her right then. I think that's how she made us all feel. She brought life and joy to every encounter.

The last visit I had with her she beamed as we walked into her room, she kept eye contact and held my hands tightly. I left her room feeling loved and encouraged, even then.

Grandma I am so thankful for you! Grateful for how you shared your love of Christ with me, your faithfulness in serving His people, and your beautiful smile as you sang songs of joy.

Letter to the Family

Dear Dick,

Hope you are all well and still enjoying your family. It has been sad to not see Thelma's smiling face as I walk into Magnolia, but her spirit still lingers in me. I was so impressed by your family and how they surrounded you and each had an essence of Thelma living in them. The recognizable smile and the loving heart that you and Thelma have passed on to them were very evident that day.

As I heard your great-granddaughter sing *Amazing Grace*, not only did the gift that God has instilled in her bring me joy it brought me to tears. I was amazed that the blood of Jesus that you believed in and surrendered yourselves to trickled its way down through generations in your family and I saw what an example of Christ you and Thelma have been to them. You have so much to be proud of and blessed by. I thought of my relationship and experience with Thelma and yourself this is what I came up with.

"Who can find a virtuous woman? For her price is far above rubies." The heart of her husband doth safely trust her… She will do him good and not evil all the days of her life… She stretcheth her hand to the poor: yea, she reacheth forth her hands to the needy. She openeth her mouth with wisdom; and in her tongue is the law of kindness. Her children arise up and call her blessed; her husband also, and he praiseth her."

Richard R. Blake

When I first met Thelma she wore denim jumpers and dresses and her hair in curls. The thing Thelma wore best was her smile. It never faded. Thelma would introduce herself as: "Hello! I am Thelma, I am a nurse, I have four sons. They are all boys." It was comical and very sweet. Thelma was very nurturing, pushing people in wheelchairs and the nurse in her trying to meet their needs whether they wanted the help or not. Many times we would let her assist walking next to a resident or holding their hand when they were upset. She was very loving. To the staff she always offered a smile and a hug. She would always tell us she loved us, regardless of the day she was having. Thelma could always be found reading her Bible even in the latter days.

When she began to decline and her loving husband, Dick, was always by her side encouraging her with words of love and strength. It was a love story acted out before our eyes.

The best memory of Thelma I will always have is how she sang with me. I would ask Thelma what song she wanted to sing and she would always name a hymn. She had several favorites and most of them were also mine. So we would sing together, never giving thought to how we sounded. Just knowing that we were singing to praise a God we both knew personally and loved. Our spirits did not know denomination, age or work they only knew we were in one accord with our same Father.

Thelma often spoke words of encouragement to me with Scripture. Whether she knew it or not or even remembered how and when, she etched a resounding mark on my heart.

156

She was created by God, I believe to be; foremost the daughter of God, the beautiful wife of Dick Blake, a mother of four amazing sons (all boys) to mold them into great men of God, a grandmother who would teach and gather those children into the love of God, a servant of God who served others, loved them all and gave the Jesus she had in her to minister and be an effective tool for Christ.

All these things that she was created to be she did with the utmost humility and love till her dying day. "Many daughters have done virtuously but thou excellest them all."

I praise God for allowing me to know Thelma and you, Dick, to minister into my life and help me to draw closer to God, because of your example. I love you both and I hope that in some small way I touched your heart, as you have not just touched me, but bulldozed me over with your kindness and love.

May God richly bless you. I plan on rejoicing with Thelma one day. I am almost sure God will have her at the pearly gates welcoming everyone with that beautiful smile of hers.

In Christ's love,
Nora Ramirez (Admission Director, Woodland Terrace Bridgman)

A Prayer of Submission
Journal Entry March 15, 2018

Father in heaven, You have given me an extra measure
of Your divine peace over the last two weeks since Jesus
took Thelma's hand and welcomed her into your
presence. We are happy for her; You have made her
whole again, replaced her fragile body, restored her
mind completely, and have given her immeasurable joy
and peace.

You have left me here to continue her legacy, to fulfill
my destiny and complete Your purpose for my life. You
have given me a blessed gift of four sons, Rick, Ken,
Jim, and Rob. Help me, Heavenly Father, to be an
instrument of healing when they suffer, and a listening
ear when they seek guidance. Make me an inspiration
and example of a man of integrity, fully devoted to
providing a legacy for them to carry on through the
families and the extended families You have given them.

Thank You for Your grace, mercy, and forgiveness, and
for the joy and peace of knowing their Mom is enjoying
the rewards of her faithfulness in honoring You
throughout her life.

Grief

My Thelma is Gone:
Journal Entry April 9, 2018

Today started out on a low note, a kind of despair. Maybe this is the beginning of a new stage of grieving. Today my purpose eluded me. My Thelma is gone. Tears dampen my cheeks as I glance at the light layer of snow accumulating on our deck, still gently falling.

Then I remembered on March 12th, one month ago, another brisk morning when snow was lightly falling, the day of Thelma's Celebration of Life service. Our extended families were meeting at the graveside for a brief service before a visitation for friends and a memorial service at the church.

As we gathered around Thelma's grave, we quietly reflected as we bonded together as a family remembering our times with Thelma. Pastor Jeff Dryden, a longtime family friend shared a few thoughts on Thelma's life. Jim Oakley, our pastor from Woodland Shores, gave us some encouraging words from the Scripture and offered up a prayer of commitment.

I quietly took note of each of our four sons, lost in personal memories of their Mom. Suddenly a beautiful burst of sunshine looked down on us, an assurance of God's pleasure at Thelma's presence in her new home.

Today, as I relived the day of the funeral with the gentle falling of snowflakes mixed with the tears on my cheeks I felt a new sense of purpose – to continue Thelma's legacy by completing the story of our journey.

"Jesus said to her, "I am the resurrection and the life. The one who believes in me will live, even though they die; And whoever lives believing in me will never die." John 11:25-26 NIV

Cherished Memories
Journal Entry April, 18, 2018

Today as I sat at my desk sorting through papers, putting together thoughts from the past, I was reminded of the wonderful gift of communication.

In her final months, even years, Thelma intuitively communicated through her eyes, facial expressions, her body language, and her smiles.

Thelma would grasp for a concept, and grapple for words, which came out in an excitement of unintelligible garble, as she sought the approval of her listener; I would attentively listen, smile my appreciation, and create conversational responses relying on my creative imagination.

Those days are over now. I cherish each memory in a renewed effort to share our story, *Our Journey with Alzheimer's*.

Questions for Reflection or Discussion

1. How can you find hope and restoration after years of caregiving?
2. How did Richard plan to keep his positive memories alive?

Letters

Bridgman, Michigan
Thursday, August 30, 2018

Dear Thelma,

I visited your grave today. I know you aren't there. I wanted to add some flowers so that others who might see them would know that we haven't forgotten your love for flowers, for pretty things, and your appreciation of the majestic beauty and splendor of God's creation.

Right now I am imagining you exploring the magnificence and grandeur of your new heavenly home; while singing praise songs to Jesus. I miss you Thelma, you gave me purpose and always supported me in my "dreams" and unfinished projects.

Each day I am blessed with family, friends, and God's rich provisions and love. We are learning from our experience with grief that we need to allow God to meet us in our sorrow and build our character. We are strengthened as we lean on Him.

Thelma, I love you,
Dick

From Thelma – At Home with the Lord

August 30, 2018

Dear Dick,

Thank you for your note. I am glad to hear you are drawing your strength from God, our Father, receiving the comfort of the Holy Spirit, and sensing the indwelling presence of Jesus.

Dick, I have to tell you about the choir here. I now have perfect pitch and a unique soprano voice that every earthly soprano would envy. A throng of us from earth join the angel choir in anthems of praise to Jesus -- truly awesome. I hope you will be blessed with a new voice when you join me someday to add your testimony of praise to our Savior and King in tribute to Him with the heavenly choir.

Jesus takes your suffering, pain and sorrow to the Father and reminds Him that He died for you. I know God will comfort you in your loneliness. Cast all your cares on Jesus instead of worrying and taking on every burden.

Thank you for the flowers, your thoughtfulness, and love. See you soon – Maybe in the next 1,000 years. Love, Thelma

Cumulative Grief

March 30, 2018, less than a month after Thelma's home going, I received a phone call telling me my brother John, a missionary in Spain, had gone to be with the Lord. In August I lost a niece. Then Thursday, November 1, 2018 another phone call. Mary, Ken's daughter was on the line. Ken had succumbed to his long battle with emphysema. I was too stunned to cry. Although I had seen evidence of the severity of his breathing problems when Ken was with me for Thelma's funeral, I had hoped this call would never come. Children are supposed to outlive their parents.

Rick arranged transportation for himself, Rob and I and a place to stay in California. My brother Dennis and sister Edna joined us there. Jim and Irma lived in the area. It was good to be there for Ken's daughters and granddaughters as we shared our grief together.

As I feel the depth of grief again, I can only imagine the reunion of Ken with his son Kenny, his mom Thelma, his uncle John and cousin Nancy who welcomed him into their presence and into the loving arms of Jesus.

Questions for Reflection or Discussion

1. How do you process grief, loss of not being able to be together?
2. What compounded Richard's grief?
3. Have you experienced multiple losses before processing your first loss? How has it affected you?
4. Richard found writing helped him process his grief. What have you found helpful?

Richard R. Blake

A Tribute of Love to my Thelma January 1, 2019

The light in your eyes lingers today.
As a sign of your warm love
Through your sparkling eyes
Your love revealed
A winning smile
Won my heart
Your smile unveils a sense of joy,
Peace but most of all, deep love
Your gentle spirit, your sparkling eyes
And a sweet smile now closed,
By death's soft hands
Now linger in my heart.
Those twinkling eyes and endearing smile
My daily smile returned.
A sign of our eternal love

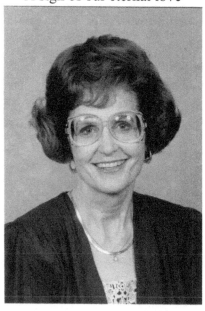

Moving On

Letter to Thelma

October 7, 2019

Dear Thelma,

It will soon be eighteen months, since the day the angels came to escort you to the heavenly realms.

Recently, I came across a moving reference from the writing of John Bunyan's book *The Pilgrims Progress*.

"It is only when Christian reaches the foot of the cross that his burdens fall off him…" but the journey doesn't end there. Bunyan goes on to describe Christian's emotions as he stood at the foot of the cross. "…inward springs of water flowed down his cheeks…"

I thought about my feelings when you left me alone with memories of our sixty-some years together. The shuddering sobs and "inward springs of water" flowing down my cheeks" have now subsided.

The sobbing has been replaced with beautiful memories of your sweet smile and gracious spirit, always supportive: always encouraging. My tears come less frequently, and the precious memories are healing the heartache.

Your smile, captured in photos on those special occasions while celebrating together, brightens nearly every room of our home. Framed pictures elicit a warm sense of celebration.

The sparkle in your eyes and the radiance of your smile triggers a response – my ongoing love for you.

Thelma, I miss you,
Dick

Two Years Later
Journal Entry March 2, 2020

Tomorrow, March 3, would have been Thelma's 85th birthday. Some exceptional memories linger in the deep caverns of my mind; however, each of the four birthdays we celebrated with our family at Woodland Terrace stand out as special.

Balloons, birthday cakes, candles, and gifts were all a part of these occasions. My princess Thelma became "Queen for a Day:" radiant, smiling, recognizing family love, though our names eluded her.

The grief process varies with individuals; although I miss Thelma very much I was amazed this morning to realize that not once yesterday, March 1, did I think back and recognize the day as the date of the second anniversary of Thelma's death.

Knick-knacks, pictures, souvenirs, books, and furniture throughout our home prompt confirmation of Thelma's influence, a kind of lasting tribute to her memory.

My love for Thelma is eternal. My grief for Thelma is, thankfully, only temporal. The raw freshness has retreated now, the pain no longer throbbing, more of an aching.

Each morning I begin the day with an inspirational time of Scripture reading accessed through the computer. Between my computer screen and a reading lamp on the desk, I have placed a framed picture of Thelma.

As I turn on the lamp, she greets me with a smile, her eyes sparkling. I still smile and may even greet her with a "Good morning, Thelma." Diminishing grief, my good morning may be delayed or forgotten until several minutes have passed when I suddenly recognize I am moving on.

Reading the Scriptures and devotional thoughts, I am reminded God has a new purpose for me. Daily, I ask Him to take my hand, guide my steps, and use me as an instrument of encouragement to the discouraged, to offer help to the hurting, and to reflect the love of Jesus in my countenance.

I am also assured Thelma has found her new purpose. She has joined the Angel Choir to sing praises to the Heavenly Father.

Richard R. Blake

The Relief and the Grief
By Edna Headland

No more calls at 4 A.M.
Saying Grandma has fallen again.

No more silly grins
with food stuck on her chin.

No more slumping asleep in her chair
while you try to wake her up to show her you care.

No more lost hearing aids, teeth, or glasses.

No more bumps, bruises, scratches or skin tears,
that appear from who knows where.

No more high blood sugars, low blood sugars
or insulin injections.

No more coaxing down one last bite
so there won't be an insulin reaction that night.

No more lying face to the wall
trying to shut out the commotion in the hall.

No more wet pads or smelly messes.

No more sweet love pats when she's all clean and dry.

No more kisses thrown in good bye.

No more eyes lit up in recognition when you appear.

No more scooting down the hall
greeting one and all.

No more "Amens" or "boo boos".

No more responses of "I love you".

No more the center of the family Christmas picture.

No more outings to the lake
for just a little ride to take.

No more shaky voice singing
along to *Trust and Obey*.

Now she is singing in perfect tune along with the saints in glory.

No more lunches choked down in the car as I rush to visit.

No more "I love yous" or hugs and kisses from other residents.

No more understanding looks or hugs
from other resident's family members who are walking the same path.

No more family council, care conferences, concern forms or visits with staff.

It has been a long four years of learning and growing. The same time it takes to earn a college degree. You have all been a part and we thank you.

End Notes

[i] https://alz.org/alzheimers-dementia/facts-figures

[ii] **The Seven Stages of Alzheimer's Disease** developed by Barry Reisberg of New York University.

Stage 1: No Impairment
During this stage, Alzheimer's is not detectable and no memory problems or other symptoms of dementia are evident.

Stage 2: Very Mild Decline
The senior may notice minor memory problems or lose things around the house, although not to the point where the memory loss can easily be distinguished from normal age-related memory loss. The person will still do well on memory tests and the disease is unlikely to be detected by loved ones or physicians.

Stage 3: Mild Decline
At this stage, the family members and friends of the senior may begin to notice cognitive problems. Performance on memory tests are affected and physicians will be able to detect impaired cognitive function.
People in stage 3 will have difficulty in many areas including:
- Finding the right word during conversations
- Organizing and planning
- Remembering names of new acquaintances

People with stage three Alzheimer's may also frequently lose personal possessions, including valuables.

Stage 4: Moderate Decline
In stage four of Alzheimer's, clear-cut symptoms of the disease are apparent. People with stage four of Alzheimer's:
- Have difficulty with simple arithmetic
- Have poor short-term memory (may not recall what they ate for breakfast, for example)
- Inability to manage finance and pay bills
- May forget details about their life histories

Stage 5: Moderately Severe Decline
During the fifth stage of Alzheimer's, people begin to need help with many day-to-day activities. People in stage five of the disease may experience:

- Difficulty dressing appropriately
- Inability to recall simple details about themselves such as their own phone number
- Significant confusion

On the other hand, people in stage five maintain functionality. They typically can still bathe and toilet independently. They also usually still know their family members and some detail about their personal histories, especially their childhood and youth.

Stage 6: Severe Decline

People with the sixth stage of Alzheimer's need constant supervision and frequently require professional care. Symptoms include:

- Confusion or unawareness of environment and surroundings
- Inability to recognize faces except for the closest friends and relatives
- Inability to remember most details of personal history
- Loss of bladder and bowel control
- Major personality changes and potential behavior problems
- The need for assistance with activities of daily living such as toileting and bathing
- Wandering

Stages 7: Very Severe Decline

Stage seven is the final stage of Alzheimer's. Because the disease is a terminal illness, people in stage seven are nearing death. In stage seven of the disease, people lose the ability to communicate or respond to their environment. While they may still be able to utter words and phrases, they have no insight into their condition and need assistance with all activities of daily living. In the final stages of Alzheimer's, people may lose their ability to swallow.